THE NATURAL HEALING HANDBOOK

SIMPLE RECIPES & REMEDIES FOR EVERY CONDITION

ANCIENT REMEDIES PRESS

Navigating the Pages

Each page is thoughtfully structured for easy reading and quick reference, featuring the following sections:

CORE HERBS

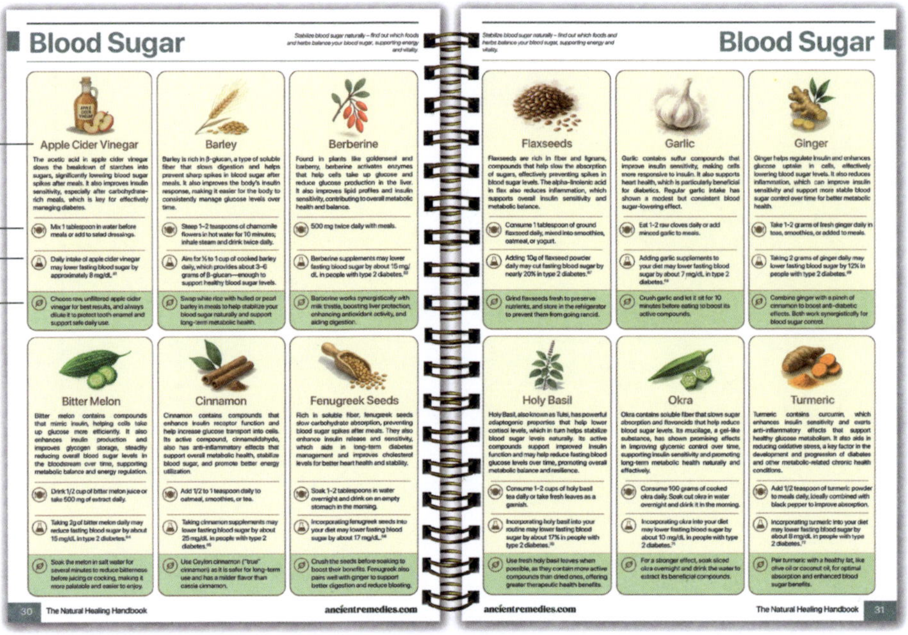

Core Herbs
Key herbs and ingredients essential for addressing the specific health condition.

Usage
General guidelines on how to incorporate the herb into daily routines.

Scientific Insights
Evidence-based studies or data supporting the effectiveness of these herbs, each linked to numbered reference sources.

Pro Tips
Handy advice to maximize the herb's benefits.

Blood Sugar

Stabilize blood sugar naturally — find out which foods and herbs balance your blood sugar, supporting energy and vitality.

Apple Cider Vinegar

The acetic acid in apple cider vinegar slows the breakdown of starches into sugars, significantly lowering blood sugar spikes after meals. It also improves insulin sensitivity, especially after carbohydrate-rich meals, which is key to effectively managing diabetes.

- Mix 1 tablespoon in water before meals or add to salad dressings.
- Daily intake of apple cider vinegar may lower fasting blood sugar by approximately 8 mg/dL.
- Choose raw, unfiltered apple cider vinegar for best results, and always dilute it to protect tooth enamel and support safe daily use.

Barley

Barley is rich in β-glucan, a type of soluble fiber that slows digestion and helps prevent sharp spikes in blood sugar after meals. It also improves the body's insulin response, making it easier for the body to consistently manage glucose levels over time.

- Steep 1–2 teaspoon of chamomile flowers in hot water for 10 minutes, inhale steam and drink twice daily.
- Aim for ¾ to 1 cup of cooked barley daily, which provides about 3–6 grams of β-glucan—enough to support healthy blood sugar levels.
- Swap white rice with hulled or pearl barley in meals to help stabilize your blood sugar naturally and support long-term metabolic health.

Berberine

Found in plants like goldenseal and barberry, berberine activates enzymes that help cells take up glucose and reduce glucose production in the liver. It also improves lipid profiles and insulin sensitivity, contributing to overall metabolic health and balance.

- 500 mg twice daily with meals.
- Berberine supplements may lower fasting blood sugar by about 15 mg/dL in people with type 2 diabetes.
- Berberine works synergistically with milk thistle, boosting liver protection, enhancing antioxidant activity, and aiding digestion.

Bitter Melon

Bitter melon contains compounds that mimic insulin, helping cells take up glucose more efficiently. It also enhances insulin production and improves glycogen storage, steadily reducing overall blood sugar levels in the bloodstream over time, supporting metabolic balance and energy regulation.

- Drink ½ cup of bitter melon juice or take 500 mg of extract daily.
- Taking 2g of bitter melon daily may reduce fasting blood sugar by about 15 mg/dL in type 2 diabetics.
- Soak the melon in salt water for several minutes to reduce bitterness before juicing or cooking, making it more palatable and easier to enjoy.

Cinnamon

Cinnamon contains compounds that enhance insulin receptor function and help increase glucose transport into cells. Its active compound, cinnamaldehyde, also has anti-inflammatory effects that support overall metabolic health, stabilize blood sugar, and promote better glucose utilization.

- Add ½ to 1 teaspoon daily to oatmeal, smoothies, or tea.
- Taking cinnamon supplements may lower fasting blood sugar by about 25 mg/dL in people with type 2 diabetes.
- Use Ceylon cinnamon ("true" cinnamon) as it is safer for long-term use and has a milder flavor than cassia cinnamon.

Fenugreek Seeds

Rich in soluble fiber, fenugreek seeds slow carbohydrate absorption, preventing blood sugar spikes after meals. They also enhance insulin release and sensitivity, which aids in long-term diabetes management and improves cholesterol levels for better heart health and stability.

- Soak 1–2 tablespoons in water overnight and drink on an empty stomach in the morning.
- Incorporating fenugreek seeds into your routine may lower fasting blood sugar by about 17 mg/dL.
- Crush the seeds before soaking to boost their benefits. Fenugreek also pairs well with ginger to support better digestion and reduce bloating.

ancientremedies.com

30 | The Natural Healing Handbook

Blood Sugar

Stabilize blood sugar naturally — find out which foods and herbs balance your blood sugar, supporting energy and vitality.

Flaxseeds

Flaxseeds are rich in fiber and lignans, compounds that help slow the absorption of sugars, effectively preventing spikes in blood sugar levels. The alpha-linolenic acid in flax also reduces inflammation, which supports overall insulin sensitivity and metabolic balance.

- Consume 1 tablespoon of ground flaxseed daily, mixed into smoothies, oatmeal, or yogurt.
- Adding 10g of flaxseed powder daily may cut fasting blood sugar by nearly 20% in type 2 diabetes.
- Grind flaxseeds fresh to preserve nutrients, and store in the refrigerator to prevent them from going rancid.

Garlic

Garlic contains sulfur compounds that improve insulin sensitivity, making cells more responsive to insulin. It also supports heart health, which is particularly beneficial for diabetics. Regular garlic intake has shown a modest but consistent blood sugar-lowering effect.

- Eat 1–2 raw cloves daily or add minced garlic to meals.
- Adding garlic supplements to your may lower fasting blood sugar by about 7 mg/dL in type 2 diabetes.
- Crush garlic and let it sit for 10 minutes before eating to boost its active compounds.

Ginger

Ginger helps regulate insulin and enhances insulin sensitivity, lowering blood sugar levels. It also reduces inflammation, which can improve insulin sensitivity and support more stable blood sugar control over time for better metabolic health.

- Take 1–2 grams of fresh ginger daily in teas, smoothies, or added to meals.
- Taking 2 grams of ginger daily may lower fasting blood sugar by 12% in people with type 2 diabetes.
- Combine ginger with a pinch of cinnamon to boost anti-diabetic effects. Both work synergistically for blood sugar control.

Holy Basil

Holy Basil, also known as Tulsi, has powerful adaptogenic properties that help lower cortisol levels, which in turn helps stabilize blood sugar levels naturally. Its active compounds support improved insulin function and may help reduce fasting blood glucose levels over time, promoting overall metabolic balance and resilience.

- Consume 1–2 cups of holy basil tea daily or take fresh leaves as a garnish.
- Incorporating holy basil into your routine may lower fasting blood sugar by about 17% in people with type 2 diabetes.
- Use fresh holy basil leaves when possible, as they contain more active compounds than dried ones, offering greater therapeutic health benefits.

Okra

Okra contains soluble fiber that slows sugar absorption and flavonoids that help reduce blood sugar levels. Its mucilage, a gel-like substance, has shown promising effects in improving glycemic control over time, supporting insulin sensitivity and promoting long-term metabolic health naturally and effectively.

- Consume 100 grams of cooked okra daily. Soak cut okra in water overnight and drink it in the morning.
- Incorporating okra into your diet may lower fasting blood sugar by about 10 mg/dL in people with type 2 diabetes.
- For a stronger effect, soak sliced okra overnight and drink the water to extract its beneficial compounds.

Turmeric

Turmeric contains curcumin, which enhances insulin sensitivity and exerts anti-inflammatory effects that support healthy glucose metabolism. It also aids in reducing oxidative stress, a key factor in the development and progression of diabetes and other metabolic-related chronic health conditions.

- Add ½ teaspoon of turmeric powder to meals daily, ideally combined with black pepper to improve absorption.
- Incorporating turmeric into your diet may lower fasting blood sugar by about 8 mg/dL in people with type 2 diabetes.
- Pair turmeric with a healthy fat, like olive oil or coconut oil, for optimal absorption and enhanced blood sugar benefits.

ancientremedies.com

The Natural Healing Handbook | 31

RECIPES

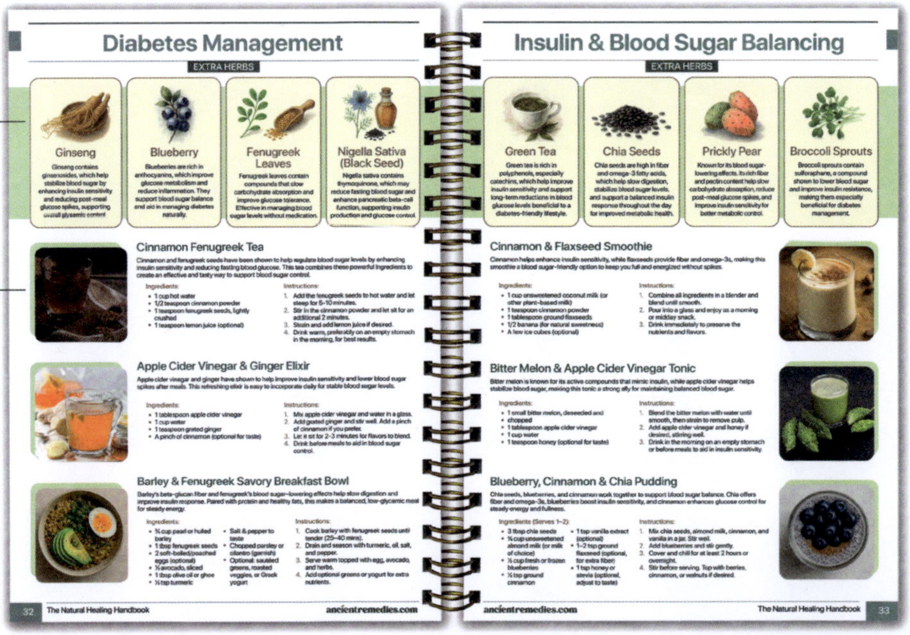

Additional Herbs
Complementary herbs that boost treatment within this specific subsection of the health condition.

Recipes
Easy-to-follow recipes that utilize both core and additional herbs to address the health condition effectively.

Diabetes Management

EXTRA HERBS

Ginseng

Ginseng contains ginsenosides, which help stabilize blood sugar by enhancing insulin sensitivity and reducing post-meal glucose spikes, supporting overall glycemic control

Blueberry

Blueberries are rich in anthocyanins, which improve glucose metabolism and reduce inflammation. They support blood sugar balance and aid in managing diabetes naturally.

Fenugreek Leaves

Fenugreek leaves contain compounds that slow carbohydrate absorption and improve glucose response. Effective in managing blood sugar levels without medication.

Nigella Sativa (Black Seed)

Nigella sativa contains thymoquinone, which may reduce fasting blood sugar and enhance pancreatic beta-cell function, supporting insulin production and glucose control.

Cinnamon Fenugreek Tea

Cinnamon and fenugreek seeds have been shown to help regulate blood sugar levels by enhancing insulin sensitivity and reducing fasting blood glucose. This tea combines these powerful ingredients to create an effective and tasty way to support blood sugar control.

Ingredients:
- 1 cup hot water
- ½ teaspoon cinnamon powder
- 1 teaspoon fenugreek seeds, lightly crushed
- 1 teaspoon lemon juice (optional)

Instructions:
1. Add the fenugreek seeds to hot water and let steep for 5–10 minutes.
2. Stir in the cinnamon powder and let sit for an additional 2 minutes.
3. Strain and add lemon juice if desired.
4. Drink warm, preferably on an empty stomach in the morning, for best results.

Apple Cider Vinegar & Ginger Elixir

Apple cider vinegar and ginger have shown to help improve insulin sensitivity and lower blood sugar spikes after meals. This refreshing elixir is easy to incorporate daily for stable blood sugar levels.

Ingredients:
- 1 tablespoon apple cider vinegar
- 1 cup water
- 1 teaspoon grated ginger
- A pinch of cinnamon (optional for taste)

Instructions:
1. Mix apple cider vinegar and water in a glass.
2. Add grated ginger and stir well. Add a pinch of cinnamon if you prefer.
3. Let it sit for 2–3 minutes for flavors to blend.
4. Drink before meals to aid in blood sugar control.

Barley & Fenugreek Savory Breakfast Bowl

Barley's beta-glucan fiber and fenugreek's blood sugar-lowering effects help slow digestion and improve insulin response. Paired with protein and healthy fats, this makes a balanced, low-glycemic meal for steady energy.

Ingredients:
- ½ cup pearl or hulled barley
- 1 tbsp fenugreek seeds
- 2 soft-boiled/poached eggs (optional)
- ¼ avocado, sliced
- 1 tbsp olive oil or ghee
- ½ tsp turmeric
- Salt & pepper to taste
- Chopped parsley or cilantro (garnish)
- Optional: sautéed greens, roasted veggies, or Greek yogurt

Instructions:
1. Cook barley with fenugreek seeds until tender (25–40 mins).
2. Drain and season with turmeric, oil, salt, and pepper.
3. Serve warm topped with egg, avocado, and herbs.
4. Add optional greens or yogurt for extra nutrients.

ancientremedies.com

32 | The Natural Healing Handbook

Insulin & Blood Sugar Balancing

EXTRA HERBS

Green Tea

Green tea is rich in polyphenols, especially catechins, which help improve insulin sensitivity and support long-term reductions in blood glucose levels beneficial to a diabetes-friendly lifestyle.

Chia Seeds

Chia seeds are high in fiber and omega-3 fatty acids, which help slow digestion, stabilize blood sugar levels, and support a balanced insulin response throughout the day for improved metabolic health.

Prickly Pear

Known for its blood sugar-lowering effects, its rich fiber and pectin content help slow carbohydrate absorption, reduce post-meal glucose spikes, and improve insulin sensitivity for better metabolic control.

Broccoli Sprouts

Broccoli sprouts contain sulforaphane, a compound shown to lower blood sugar and improve insulin resistance, making them especially beneficial for diabetes management.

Cinnamon & Flaxseed Smoothie

Cinnamon helps enhance insulin sensitivity, while flaxseeds provide fiber and omega-3s, making this smoothie a blood sugar-friendly option to keep you full and energized without spikes.

Ingredients:
- 1 cup unsweetened coconut milk (or other plant-based milk)
- 1 teaspoon cinnamon powder
- 1 tablespoon ground flaxseeds
- ½ banana (for natural sweetness)
- A few ice cubes (optional)

Instructions:
1. Combine all ingredients in a blender and blend until smooth.
2. Pour into a glass and enjoy as a morning or midday snack.
3. Drink immediately to preserve the nutrients and flavors.

Bitter Melon & Apple Cider Vinegar Tonic

Bitter melon is known for its active compounds that mimic insulin, while apple cider vinegar helps stabilize blood sugar, making this tonic a strong ally for maintaining balanced blood sugar.

Ingredients:
- 1 small bitter melon, deseeded and chopped
- 1 tablespoon apple cider vinegar
- 1 cup water
- 1 teaspoon honey (optional for taste)

Instructions:
1. Blend the bitter melon with water until smooth, then strain to remove pulp.
2. Add apple cider vinegar and honey if desired, stirring well.
3. Drink in the morning on an empty stomach or before meals to aid in insulin sensitivity.

Blueberry, Cinnamon & Chia Pudding

Chia seeds, blueberries, and cinnamon work together to support blood sugar balance. Chia offers fiber and omega-3s, blueberries boost insulin sensitivity, and cinnamon enhances glucose control for steady energy and fullness.

Ingredients (Serves 1–2):
- 3 tbsp chia seeds
- ½ cup unsweetened almond milk (or milk of choice)
- ¼ cup fresh or frozen blueberries
- ½ tsp ground cinnamon
- 1 tsp vanilla extract (optional)
- 1–2 tsp ground flaxseed (optional, for extra fiber)
- 1 tsp honey or stevia (optional, adjust to taste)

Instructions:
1. Mix chia seeds, almond milk, cinnamon, and vanilla in a jar. Stir well.
2. Add blueberries and stir gently.
3. Cover and chill for at least 2 hours or overnight.
4. Stir before serving. Top with berries, cinnamon, or walnuts if desired.

ancientremedies.com

The Natural Healing Handbook | 33

To access the full list of all the scientific insights, go to https://ancientremedies.com/pages/nhhreferences

Introduction

At Ancient Remedies, we believe that true healing comes from aligning the wisdom of nature with the needs of modern life. Founded on the timeless principles of holistic wellness, our mission is to revive and share the ancient practices that have supported human health for centuries, empowering people to take control of their well-being through natural, time-tested methods.

We are dedicated to providing trusted, research-based resources that illuminate the power of traditional medicine. Drawing from systems like Traditional Chinese Medicine, Ayurveda, and other holistic practices from around the world, we explore how these age-old remedies can support the mind, body, and spirit in today's fast-paced world. Our content is designed to be accessible, informative, and actionable—bridging the gap between ancient insight and modern wellness.

The Natural Healing Handbook is designed to support you in integrating these principles into your daily life and exploring the deep knowledge passed down through generations of remedies that nourished the body, calmed the mind, and strengthened the spirit long before modern medicine emerged. Whether you're new to holistic health or deepening an existing practice, this book offers practical tools, trusted remedies, and empowering routines to help you take charge of your well-being.

Before we delve into the practical tools and remedies that await you, let's begin by clarifying some key terms and concepts that will guide our exploration of holistic wellness and natural healing practices.

- **Free Radical:** Unstable molecules that can damage cells, contributing to aging and diseases.
- **Antioxidant:** A substance that protects cells from damage caused by free radicals.
- **Oxidative Stress:** An imbalance between free radicals and antioxidants, leading to cell damage.
- **Inflammation:** The body's response to injury or infection, often causing redness, heat, and pain.
- **Polyphenol:** Plant compounds with antioxidant properties, helping protect cells from damage.
- **Flavonoid:** A group of antioxidants found in plants, supporting heart and brain health.
- **Nitric Oxide:** A molecule that helps relax blood vessels, improving blood flow and circulation.
- **Diuretic:** A substance that increases urine production, helping reduce fluid retention in the body.
- **Adaptogen:** A natural substance that helps the body adapt to stress and restore balance.
- **Neuron:** A nerve cell that transmits electrical signals in the brain and nervous system.
- **Antimicrobial:** A substance that kills or inhibits the growth of microorganisms, such as bacteria or fungi.
- **Insulin Sensitivity:** The body's ability to respond to insulin effectively, aiding in blood sugar regulation.
- **Thermogenesis:** The process of generating heat in the body, often related to fat metabolism.

Your Wellness Guide

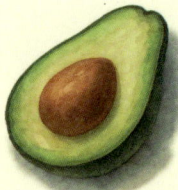

Heart Health

Nourish your heart naturally—discover herbs and foods that protect, strengthen, and energize your most vital organ from within.

Avocado

Avocados are rich in monounsaturated fats, potassium, and fiber, which help lower LDL cholesterol, reduce inflammation, and support heart function. Their potassium content also helps regulate blood pressure by balancing sodium levels and promoting overall cardiovascular health.

Aim for ½ avocado daily, on toast, in salads, or as a dip.

Eating avocados may raise HDL ('good') cholesterol by about 3 mg/dL, supporting heart and circulation health.[1]

Avocado oil is ideal for cooking, as it retains heart-healthy fats and nutrients when used at moderate heat levels.

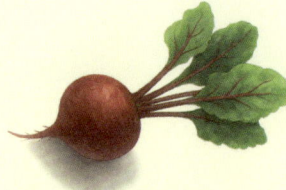

Beetroot

Beetroot is high in dietary nitrates, which are converted to nitric oxide in the body, helping to relax blood vessels and improve blood flow. This reduces blood pressure and supports overall cardiovascular health. The antioxidants in beetroot also combat inflammation.

Drink 1 cup (250 ml) of fresh beet juice or eat ½ cup cooked beetroot daily.

Drinking beetroot juice may lower systolic blood pressure by about 4 mmHg and diastolic by 1 mmHg.[2]

Consume raw or lightly cooked beets to maximize nitrate content and support optimal circulation and heart health.

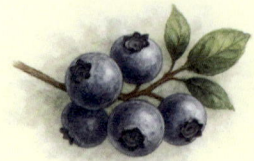

Blueberries

Berries are rich in polyphenols, including anthocyanins, which help widen blood vessels and improve circulation. They support heart health by lowering LDL cholesterol and reducing oxidative stress. Their high antioxidant content helps reduce inflammation in arteries.

Eat 1 cup of fresh or frozen berries daily.

Blueberries may lower LDL by 5 mg/dL, cut triglycerides by 6 mg/dL, and raise HDL by 11 mg/dL.[3]

Mix with strawberries, blackberries, or other berries to boost flavor and increase your intake of diverse, powerful antioxidants naturally.

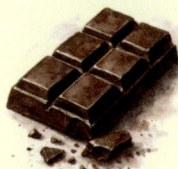

Dark Chocolate

Dark chocolate is rich in flavonoids, specifically epicatechin, which promotes the production of nitric oxide. This relaxes blood vessels, enhancing blood flow and lowering blood pressure. It also has antioxidant properties that protect the heart by reducing oxidative stress and inflammation.

Enjoy 1–2 small squares (20–30 g) of dark chocolate per day.

Eating 45 g of dark chocolate weekly may reduce cardiovascular disease risk by 11%.[4]

Choose chocolate with at least 70% cocoa for the best heart-protective benefits.

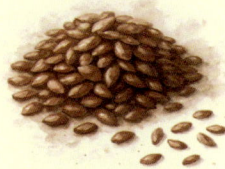

Flaxseeds

Flaxseeds are packed with omega-3 fatty acids, lignans, and soluble fiber. Together, these nutrients help lower LDL cholesterol, ease arterial inflammation, and support healthy blood pressure. They also bind to cholesterol in the gut, aiding in its removal and promoting overall cardiovascular health and balance.

Add 1–2 tablespoons of ground flaxseeds to smoothies, oatmeal, or yogurt daily.

Flaxseed can help drop total cholesterol by 12, cut LDL by 10, and slash triglycerides by 20 mg/dL.[5]

Always grind flaxseeds before eating to absorb nutrients—store in the fridge to keep them fresh.

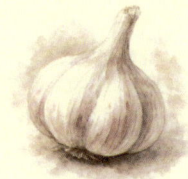

Garlic

Garlic contains allicin, a sulfur compound known to widen blood vessels, enhancing blood flow and reducing hypertension. It lowers LDL cholesterol by limiting cholesterol synthesis in the liver and helps prevent atherosclerosis with its anti-inflammatory properties and antioxidant protective effects.

Consume 1–2 raw cloves daily or add minced garlic to meals.

Garlic supplements may reduce blood pressure by about 8 mmHg systolic and 5 mmHg diastolic.[6]

Chop or crush garlic and let it sit for 10 minutes before using to maximize allicin production and health benefits.

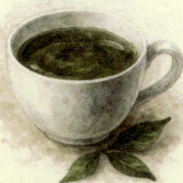

Nourish your heart naturally—discover herbs and foods that protect, strengthen, and energize your most vital organ from within.

Heart Health

Green Tea

Green tea is rich in catechins, particularly EGCG, which enhance blood vessel function and reduce LDL oxidation. Its antioxidant properties help protect against arterial damage and improve cholesterol ratios by raising HDL levels.

- Drink 2-3 cups of green tea daily for optimal benefits.

- Daily green tea consumption may lower the risk of dying from cardiovascular diseases by up to 33%.[7]

- Steep tea for 3–4 minutes, then add lemon to enhance flavor and increase antioxidant absorption by up to four times.

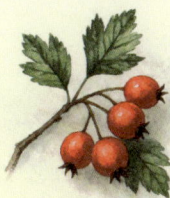

Hawthorn Berry

Hawthorn berries are rich in flavonoids and procyanidins that strengthen heart muscle contraction, dilate blood vessels, and increase blood flow. These properties help maintain stable blood pressure and reduce the risk of heart failure.

- Take 250–500 mg extract or drink hawthorn tea twice daily.

- Taking 900 mg of hawthorn extract daily may reduce the risk of sudden cardiac death in heart failure patients.[8]

- Best consumed as a tea or tincture; combining with vitamin C-rich foods may enhance nutrient absorption and overall effectiveness.

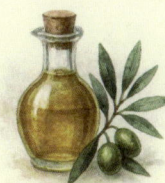

Olive Oil

Olive oil is rich in monounsaturated fats and powerful antioxidants like oleuropein and hydroxytyrosol, which help reduce oxidative damage and protect arterial walls. Its phenolic compounds support flexible, healthy blood vessels and enhance HDL (good) cholesterol levels, making it a staple for heart health.

- Use 1-2 tablespoons of extra virgin olive oil per day in cooking or drizzled on food.

- Just 10 g of olive oil daily may reduce heart disease risk by 7% and overall mortality risk by 8%.[9]

- Store in a cool, dark place to preserve its antioxidant properties and avoid refined varieties for maximum benefits.

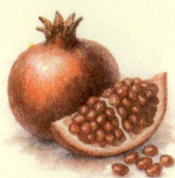

Pomegranate

Pomegranates are rich in polyphenols and antioxidants that support blood vessel health and enhance circulation. They help prevent the oxidation of LDL cholesterol, reducing arterial plaque buildup. Drinking pomegranate juice has also been linked to lower systolic blood pressure and improved overall heart function.

- Drink 1 cup (250 mL) of fresh pomegranate juice or eat 1/2 cup of seeds daily.

- Drinking pomegranate juice may lower systolic blood pressure by approximately 5 mmHg and diastolic blood pressure by about 2 mmHg.[10]

- Choose fresh 100% juice with no added sugars to maximize health benefits and avoid unnecessary spikes in blood sugar.

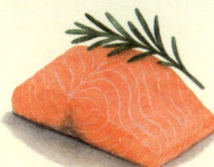

Salmon

Fatty fish are packed with heart-healthy omega-3 fatty acids, especially EPA and DHA. These essential fats help lower inflammation throughout the body, improve the health and flexibility of blood vessels, and reduce the risk of plaque buildup, supporting overall cardiovascular function and long-term heart health.

- Eat two servings per week (about 100 g cooked per serving) to support cardiovascular health.

- Fatty fish consumption lowers the risk of coronary heart disease, CHD-related death, and overall mortality.[11]

- Season with lemon, garlic, or herbs for flavor—bake or grill instead of frying to preserve heart-healthy fats.

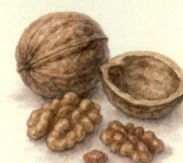

Walnuts

Walnuts are loaded with omega-3 fatty acids, antioxidants, and L-arginine, an amino acid that boosts nitric oxide production. Together, these nutrients help reduce LDL cholesterol, lower inflammation in the arteries, and promote blood vessel relaxation, improving circulation and supporting overall cardiovascular health.

- Eat a handful (about 1 ounce) of raw, unsalted walnuts daily.

- Adding walnuts to your diet may help lower total cholesterol by 3.25% and LDL (bad) cholesterol by 3.73%.[12]

- Soak walnuts overnight to boost nutrient absorption, improve digestion, and reduce compounds that may hinder mineral uptake.

Heart Function & Circulation

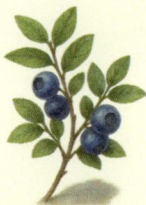

Bilberry

Rich in anthocyanins, bilberry enhances circulation, boosts eye health, and strengthens vessel walls. Clinical studies have linked it to better vascular function and improved capillary integrity.

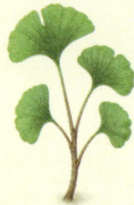

Ginkgo Biloba

Containing flavonoids and terpenoids, ginkgo biloba improves circulation and oxygen delivery by dilating vessels. It's well-studied for its vascular benefits, though slightly less common.

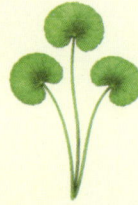

Gotu Kola

Gotu kola promotes healthy circulation by strengthening small blood vessels and easing fluid buildup. Traditionally, it's used to reduce swelling, boost vein health, and improve blood flow in the legs.

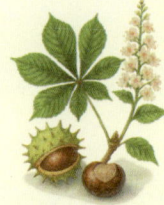

Horse Chestnut

Known for enhancing blood flow and strengthening veins, horse chestnut contains aescin, which boosts circulation, reduces swelling, and fortifies blood vessel walls.

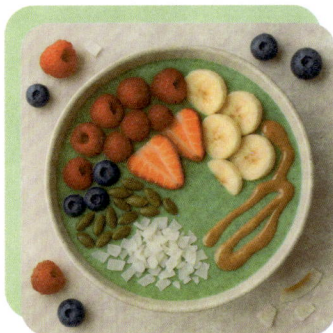

Spirulina & Berry Smoothie Bowl

This vibrant smoothie bowl is powered by spirulina, a nutrient-rich blue-green algae loaded with antioxidants, protein, iron, and anti-inflammatory compounds. Paired with berries, which are rich in anthocyanins and polyphenols, it supports heart health, boosts energy, and promotes detoxification.

Ingredients (1 Serving):

- 1 cup frozen mixed berries (e.g. blueberries, raspberries, strawberries)
- ½ frozen banana (for creaminess)
- ½ to 1 tsp spirulina powder
- 1 tbsp ground flaxseeds (optional, for omega-3s and fiber)
- ½ cup unsweetened plant milk or coconut water (adjust for thickness)

Instructions:

1. Blend all smoothie ingredients until thick and creamy. Use a tamper or stop to scrape down as needed.
2. Pour into a bowl and smooth out the top.
3. Add your favorite toppings for crunch, color, and extra nutrition.
4. Serve immediately with a spoon and enjoy.

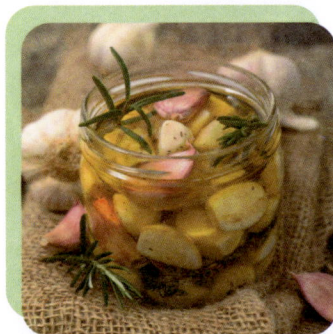

Garlic & Rosemary Infused Olive Oil Drizzle

This simple yet powerful infused oil combines garlic and rosemary to boost heart function and circulation. Garlic supports vascular health and circulation, while rosemary stimulates the cardiovascular system for enhanced blood flow.

Ingredients:

- 1/2 cup extra virgin olive oil
- 3 cloves garlic, thinly sliced
- 2 sprigs of fresh rosemary

Instructions:

1. Gently heat olive oil in a small saucepan over low heat.
2. Add garlic and rosemary; simmer gently for 10 minutes without boiling.
3. Remove from heat and let cool. Strain and store in a glass jar.
4. Drizzle on salads, veggies, or bread for a heart-healthy boost.

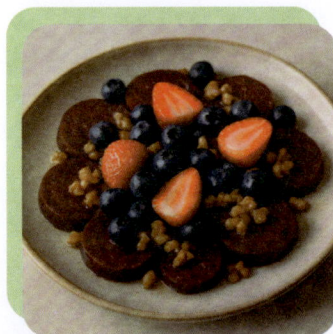

Berry & Beet Salad with Walnuts

This vibrant salad combines beets, walnuts, and berries for a dish rich in nitrates, antioxidants, and healthy fats. Beets help improve circulation, while walnuts and berries add heart-supportive nutrients for a delicious, nutrient-dense meal.

Ingredients:

- 1 medium beet, roasted and sliced
- 1/2 cup mixed berries (e.g., strawberries and blueberries)
- 1/4 cup walnuts, chopped
- 1 tbsp lemon juice
- 1 tbsp olive oil

Instructions:

1. Roast 1 medium beet, then peel and slice it.
2. Arrange beet slices with ½ cup mixed berries and ¼ cup chopped walnuts.
3. Whisk together 1 tablespoon lemon juice and 1 tablespoon olive oil.
4. Drizzle the dressing over the salad.
5. Serve immediately or chill slightly before serving.

Blood Pressure

EXTRA HERBS

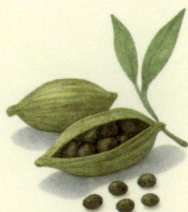

Cardamom

Cardamom is known for its powerful antioxidant, anti-inflammatory, digestive, and mild diuretic effects. Clinical trials show it can help naturally lower blood pressure in people with elevated levels.

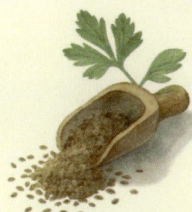

Celery Seed

Celery seed contains phthalides, which relax artery walls, reduce inflammation, and improve blood flow, thereby reducing blood pressure. Studies support its role in managing hypertension.

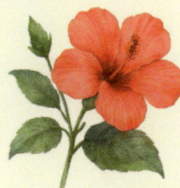

Hibiscus

Hibiscus tea has been shown to significantly lower blood pressure due to its diuretic natural effects, high antioxidant and anthocyanin content, and its ability to reduce inflammation and improve circulation.

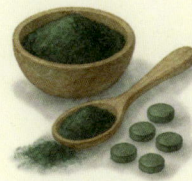

Spirulina

Spirulina is rich in antioxidants that relax blood vessels, reduce inflammation, and enhance circulation. It also provides potassium and magnesium, which support healthy blood pressure and heart function.

Hibiscus & Lemon Heart Tonic

This blend of hibiscus and lemon, both renowned for reducing blood pressure, combines heart-supporting anthocyanins from hibiscus with the vascular benefits of lemon's vitamin C and flavonoids to enhance circulation.

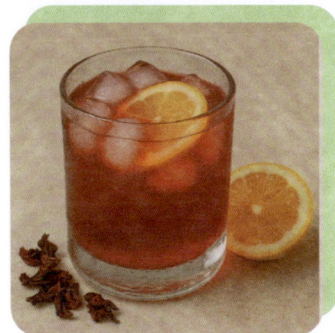

Ingredients:
- 1 tbsp dried hibiscus petals
- 1 tsp freshly squeezed lemon juice
- 1 tsp honey (optional for taste)
- 2 cups water

Instructions:
1. Boil 2 cups of water and add the dried hibiscus petals.
2. Let steep for 10 minutes, then strain the liquid into a glass.
3. Stir in the lemon juice and honey.
4. Serve warm or chilled over ice for a refreshing heart-healthy drink.

Beetroot & Ginger Smoothie

This smoothie leverages beetroot's natural nitrates and ginger's anti-inflammatory properties to promote vasodilation and reduce blood pressure. It's a vibrant, energizing drink that's as good for your taste buds as it is for your heart.

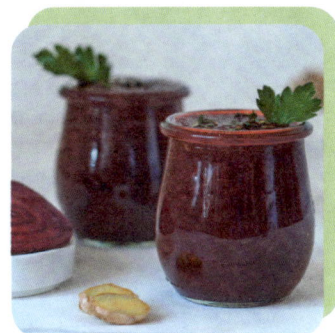

Ingredients:
- 1 small beetroot, peeled and chopped
- 1/2 inch fresh ginger root, peeled
- 1/2 cup fresh spinach leaves
- 1 cup water or coconut water
- 1 tbsp lemon juice

Instructions:
1. Add the beetroot, ginger, spinach, and water to a blender.
2. Blend until smooth and add the lemon juice.
3. Pour into a glass and serve immediately.

Pan-Seared Salmon with Cardamom-Citrus Glaze

Salmon is rich in omega-3 fatty acids, crucial for hormone production, cardiovascular health, and reducing inflammation. Cardamom supports circulation and may improve sexual function and antioxidant status.

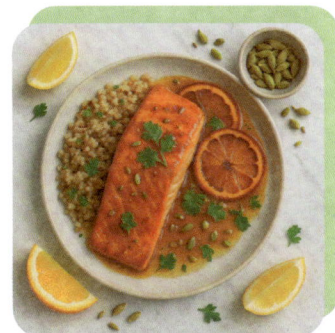

Ingredients:
- 2 salmon fillets (about 5–6 oz each)
- 1 tbsp olive oil or ghee
- Juice of ½ orange
- 1 tsp orange zest
- ½ tsp ground cardamom
- 1 tbsp honey

Instructions:
1. Mix orange juice, zest, honey, and cardamom in a bowl. Set aside.
2. Heat oil in a skillet. Cook salmon skin-side down for 4–5 mins, then flip and cook 2–3 mins more.
3. Pour glaze over salmon in the last 1–2 mins to let it reduce and coat.

Cholesterol Management

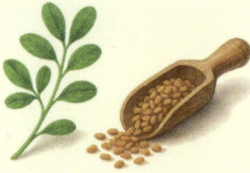

Fenugreek

Fenugreek contains soluble fiber, which effectively lowers LDL cholesterol by interfering with bile absorption in the intestines. Studies support its beneficial effects when taken regularly.

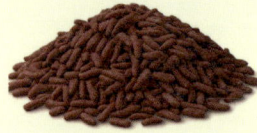

Red Yeast Rice

Red yeast rice contains monacolin K, a compound similar to statins used in cholesterol drugs. Clinical trials show it effectively lowers LDL cholesterol levels safely and naturally.

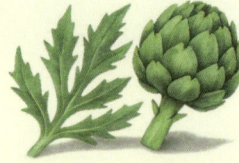

Artichoke Leaf

Artichoke leaf stimulates bile production, aiding cholesterol breakdown, improving fat digestion, and lowering LDL. Research supports its use for improving overall lipid profiles and heart health.

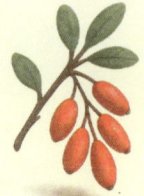

Berberine

Berberine, found in plants like barberry, helps reduce LDL ("bad") cholesterol by improving fat metabolism in the liver, enhancing insulin sensitivity, and supporting heart health.

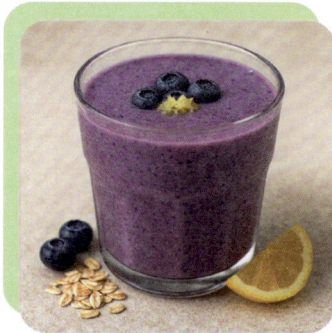

Heart-Healthy Smoothie

This smoothie leverages the cholesterol-lowering power of oats and flaxseeds combined with the antioxidant benefits of berries and the anti-inflammatory properties of ginger. This combination is designed to help manage cholesterol levels and promote overall heart health.

Ingredients:

- 1/2 cup rolled oats
- 1 tbsp flaxseeds
- 1/2 cup blueberries
- 1/2 tsp grated fresh ginger
- 1 cup almond milk (unsweetened)

Instructions:

1. Soak the oats in almond milk for 10 minutes to soften.
2. Add all ingredients to a blender and blend until smooth.
3. Pour into a glass and enjoy this nutrient-packed, cholesterol-lowering smoothie in the morning or as an afternoon snack.

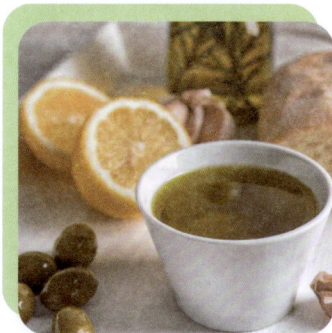

Lemon-Garlic Infused Olive Oil Dip

Combining the cholesterol-lowering effects of garlic and olive oil with the cleansing properties of lemon, this easy-to-make dip is perfect for promoting healthy cholesterol levels when used as a bread dip or salad dressing.

Ingredients:

- 1/4 cup extra virgin olive oil
- 2 cloves garlic, minced
- 1 tbsp fresh lemon juice
- A pinch of black pepper
- A sprinkle of parsley (optional for garnish)

Instructions:

1. Combine the olive oil, minced garlic, lemon juice, and black pepper in a small bowl.
2. Mix well and let the mixture sit for 10-15 minutes to infuse the flavors.
3. Serve as a dip for whole grain bread or drizzle over salads for a heart-healthy dressing.

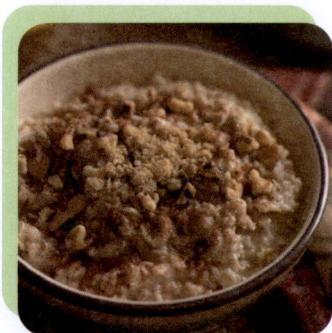

Spiced Cinnamon Oatmeal

Oats and cinnamon both help lower cholesterol levels, making this a delicious and effective breakfast option. Adding walnuts boosts the recipe's omega-3 content, which is also beneficial for heart health.

Ingredients:

- 1/2 cup rolled oats
- 1 cup water or unsweetened almond milk
- 1/2 tsp cinnamon
- 1 tbsp chopped walnuts
- 1 tsp honey or maple syrup (optional)

Instructions:

1. Bring the water or almond milk to a boil and stir in the oats.
2. Reduce the heat and let the oats simmer for about 5 minutes, stirring occasionally.
3. Add the cinnamon and chopped walnuts, stirring to combine.
4. Sweeten with honey or maple syrup if desired. Serve warm for a satisfying, heart-healthy start to your day.

Inflammation Reduction

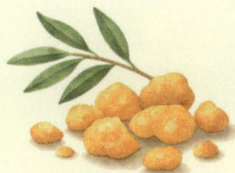

Boswellia

Boswellia contains boswellic acids, which are strong anti-inflammatory agents that block pro-inflammatory enzymes. It's commonly used to reduce chronic inflammation linked to heart issues.

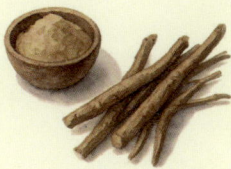

Ashwagandha

Ashwagandha is known for its powerful adaptogenic effects, helping reduce stress, balance hormones, and lower systemic inflammation. Research shows it lowers inflammatory markers like C-reactive protein (CRP).

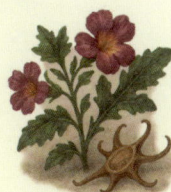

Devil's Claw

Devil's claw contains iridoid glycosides, powerful anti-inflammatory compounds. It's widely used in herbal medicine to ease inflammation and relieve pain naturally.

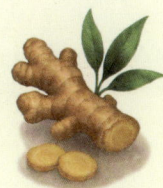

Ginger

Ginger has gingerol and shogaol, compounds that reduce inflammation by blocking harmful proteins. It helps prevent plaque buildup and supports overall heart health.

Turmeric & Ginger Anti-Inflammatory Tea

This soothing tea combines turmeric and ginger, two potent anti-inflammatory agents that can help reduce chronic inflammation and promote heart health. The addition of lemon and honey boosts its antioxidant properties and makes it deliciously refreshing.

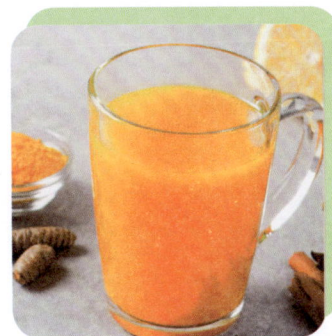

Ingredients:
- 1 tsp of ground turmeric (or 1-inch fresh turmeric root, grated)
- 1 tsp of grated fresh ginger
- 1 tbsp of lemon juice
- 1 tsp of honey (optional)
- 2 cups of water

Instructions:
1. Bring the water to a boil in a small pot.
2. Add the grated ginger and turmeric and reduce the heat to a simmer.
3. Let it simmer for 10 minutes.
4. Strain the tea into a mug, add the lemon juice and honey, and stir well.
5. Enjoy warm for maximum benefits.

Spiced Beetroot and Walnut Salad

This hearty salad features beets, walnuts, and olive oil, all of which are known to reduce inflammation. The beets provide nitrates for improved circulation, while walnuts and olive oil offer anti-inflammatory omega-3s.

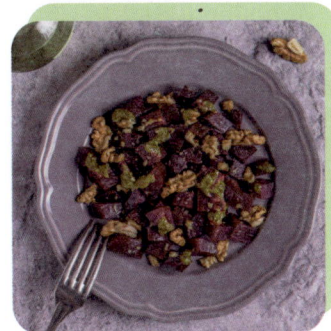

Ingredients:
- 2 medium-sized beetroots, roasted and diced
- 1/3 cup of chopped walnuts
- 2 tbsp of extra-virgin olive oil
- 1 tbsp of apple cider vinegar
- Salt and black pepper to taste

Instructions:
1. Roast the beetroots at 400°F (200°C) for 45 minutes or until tender. Let them cool and dice into cubes.
2. In a large bowl, combine the diced beetroot, walnuts, olive oil, and apple cider vinegar.
3. Season with salt and black pepper to taste and toss well.
4. Serve as a side dish or light meal.

Golden Milk with Cinnamon and Cardamom

This classic golden milk recipe uses the anti-inflammatory power of turmeric combined with cinnamon and cardamom to create a warm, comforting drink that soothes inflammation and promotes heart health.

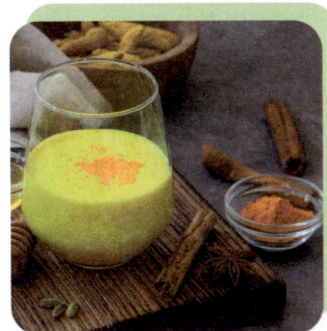

Ingredients:
- 1 cup of unsweetened almond milk (or preferred milk)
- 1/2 tsp of ground turmeric
- 1/4 tsp of ground cinnamon
- 1/4 tsp of ground cardamom
- 1 tsp of honey or maple syrup (optional)
- A pinch of black pepper (to enhance turmeric absorption)

Instructions:
1. Heat the almond milk in a small saucepan over medium heat.
2. Add the turmeric, cinnamon, cardamom, and black pepper. Whisk continuously for 3-5 minutes until warm but not boiling.
3. Remove from heat and stir in the honey or maple syrup, if desired.
4. Pour into a mug and enjoy warm.

Brain Health

Boost your brainpower naturally – explore foods and herbs that enhance cognition, focus, and mental clarity from within.

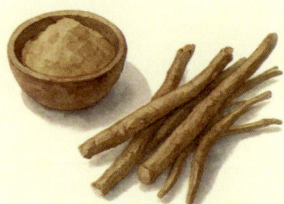

Ashwagandha

Ashwagandha, an adaptogenic herb, helps lower cortisol levels, which mitigates stress and promotes mental clarity. Its active compounds, withanolides, support neuron health, enhance memory, and reduce cognitive decline. It boosts brain function by protecting nerve cells from free radicals.

- Take 300–500 mg of standardized root extract daily, or brew 1 teaspoon dried root in hot water as tea.

- Taking 300 mg twice daily for 8 weeks improved memory by 28% in adults with mild cognitive impairment.[13]

- Pair with warm milk for better absorption and enhanced soothing nighttime benefits.

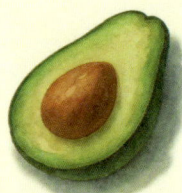

Avocado

Avocados are rich in monounsaturated fats, which promote blood flow and support brain health. They contain lutein, shown to improve cognitive performance, and is a source of antioxidants. Regular consumption supports attention and memory over time.

- Consume half an avocado daily in salads or as a spread.

- Eating avocado or guacamole may boost immediate word recall by 15% in older adults.[14]

- Combine with leafy greens to maximize lutein absorption and cognitive benefits.

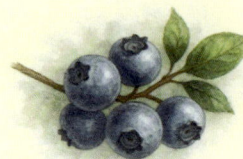

Blueberries

Blueberries are packed with antioxidants, especially flavonoids, which combat oxidative stress and inflammation in the brain. This enhances communication between brain cells and improves overall cognitive function. They are linked to better long-term memory and clearer thinking.

- Eat ½ cup of fresh or frozen berries daily.

- 26 g of freeze-dried wild blueberries daily for 12 weeks improved memory and attention in older adults.[15]

- Pair with nuts or seeds rich in omega-3s to boost cognitive benefits and support brain function.

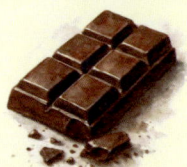

Dark Chocolate

Dark chocolate contains flavonoids that enhance blood flow to the brain, promoting cognitive function, sharpening focus, and reducing mental fatigue. The magnesium content helps with relaxation and mood stabilization, supporting overall mental health, emotional balance, and stress resilience.

- Enjoy 1–2 squares (20–30 g) of 70% or higher dark chocolate a few times a week.

- 35 g of high-flavanol chocolate improved visual attention and mental performance.[16]

- Choose dark chocolate with minimal added sugar and high cocoa content.

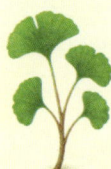

Ginkgo biloba

Ginkgo Biloba contains terpenoids and flavonoids that increase blood circulation and protect brain cells from oxidative damage. This enhanced blood flow supports memory retention, mental clarity, and concentration, particularly in aging adults and those with cognitive decline or memory loss.

- Take 120–240 mg of standardized ginkgo biloba extract per day, split into two doses.

- 240 mg of Ginkgo biloba extract daily for 24 weeks may improve cognition in mild cognitive impairment.[17]

- Combine with foods rich in omega-3 fatty acids for a synergistic effect on brain health.

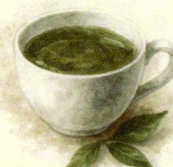

Green Tea

Green tea contains both L-theanine and caffeine, which together promote alertness without the jitters. L-theanine increases alpha brain wave activity, fostering a state of relaxed focus, reducing mental fatigue, boosting learning ability, and improving overall cognitive function and clarity.

- Drink 2–3 cups of green tea daily for optimal benefits.

- Drinking green tea daily may lower the risk of cognitive decline by 36%.[18]

- Brew for 2–3 minutes to maximize L-theanine content and flavor. Pair with a slice of lemon to enhance antioxidant absorption.

Boost your brainpower naturally – explore foods and herbs that enhance cognition, focus, and mental clarity from within.

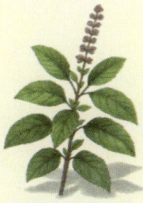

Holy Basil (Tulsi)

Holy Basil, or Tulsi, is an adaptogenic herb that helps manage stress by balancing cortisol and enhancing resilience. Its antioxidants protect brain cells, supporting memory, mood, and mental clarity. Holy Basil also reduces anxiety and boosts focus, especially under stress.

- Brew 1–2 teaspoons of dried leaves in hot water for a calming tea.

- Taking 300 mg of holy basil extract daily for 15 days improved short-term memory and focus.[19]

- Try with a creamy milk alternative for a soothing, stress-relieving drink before bedtime.

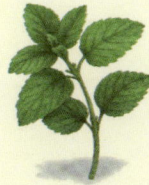

Lemon Balm

Lemon balm contains rosmarinic acid, which increases GABA levels in the brain, promoting relaxation and reducing overactivity. It helps boost memory and cognitive performance through its antioxidant properties. It is known for reducing stress-induced cognitive decline.

- Steep 1–2 teaspoons of dried lemon balm leaves in hot water for 10 minutes. Drink up to 3 times daily.

- 600 mg of lemon balm extract daily for 4 months may improve cognition in mild to moderate Alzheimer's.[20]

- Combine with chamomile tea for enhanced relaxation effects and flavor.

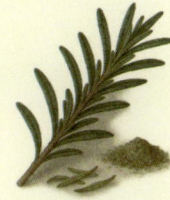

Rosemary

Rosemary contains carnosic acid and 1,8-cineole, compounds that stimulate brain function by increasing cerebral blood flow and protecting neurons from oxidative damage. It supports long-term brain health and boosts recall and accuracy during mental tasks.

- Inhale rosemary oil for 5–10 minutes or add 1 teaspoon of dried rosemary leaves to hot water for tea.

- Consuming 750 mg of dried rosemary powder may enhance memory speed in older adults.[21]

- Pair rosemary with lemon balm tea for synergistic brain-boosting effects and a delightful taste.

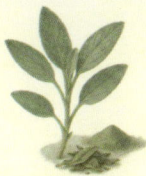

Sage

Sage contains active compounds such as rosmarinic acid and antioxidants that improve cognitive performance by protecting neurons from oxidative stress and supporting neurotransmitter activity. Studies have shown that sage extracts boost acetylcholine levels, vital for memory and learning.

- Brew 1–2 teaspoons of dried sage leaves in hot water for tea or add fresh leaves to meals.

- Taking 333 mg of sage extract may enhance memory and attention in healthy older adults.[22]

- Fresh sage can be steeped in oil to create a brain-boosting infusion for salads and light dishes.

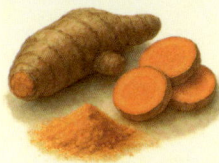

Turmeric

Curcumin, the main active compound in turmeric, crosses the blood-brain barrier and combats inflammation and oxidative damage. It boosts brain-derived neurotrophic factor, supporting neuron growth, mental sharpness, emotional balance, memory retention, and overall brain health and longevity.

- Consume ¼ teaspoon of turmeric powder with a pinch of black pepper daily for optimal absorption.

- 90 mg of curcumin twice daily for 18 months may boost memory by 28% in older adults with mild memory issues.[23]

- Pair turmeric with blueberries to combine its anti-inflammatory benefits with antioxidants, protecting brain cells from oxidative stress.

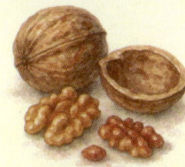

Walnuts

Walnuts are rich in alpha-linolenic acid and polyphenols that protect brain cells, reduce inflammation, and support mood. They also contain DHA, an omega-3 fatty acid linked to improved brain function and neuroprotection. Regular walnut intake enhances processing, memory, and cognition.

- Consume a handful (about 1 ounce) of walnuts daily as a snack or add to salads and cereals.

- Approximately 10 grams of walnuts daily may enhance cognitive functions like reaction time and memory.[24]

- Soak walnuts overnight for better nutrient absorption, easier digestion, and a smoother taste.

Memory & Cognitive Function

EXTRA HERBS

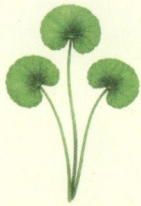

Gotu Kola

Gotu kola has a long history in traditional medicine for enhancing memory and cognition. Studies suggest it boosts brain circulation and improves processing speed and recall.

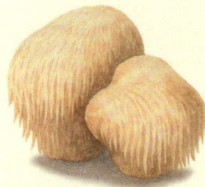

Lion's Mane

Lion's mane mushroom increases nerve growth factor, which is vital for neuron health. Clinical trials show it may improve mild cognitive impairment, support memory function, and enhance mental clarity.

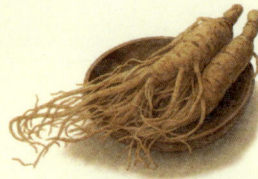

Panax Ginseng

Panax ginseng is known for its cognitive-enhancing effects, including improved memory, learning, and mental performance. Studies show benefits across all age groups, both young and old.

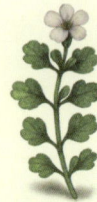

Brahmi

Brahmi (Bacopa monnieri), used in Ayurvedic medicine, improves cognition by enhancing nerve transmission and increasing acetylcholine, a key chemical for learning and memory.

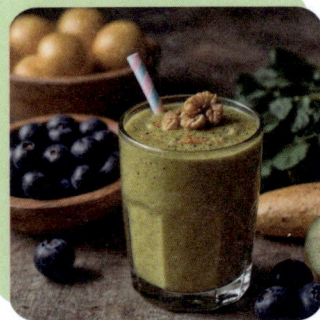

Golden Memory Boost Smoothie

This smoothie blends turmeric, blueberries, spinach, and walnuts to boost memory and brain health by reducing inflammation, improving blood flow, and protecting against oxidative stress.

Ingredients:

- 1 tsp turmeric powder (with a pinch of black pepper for absorption)
- 1 cup fresh or frozen blueberries
- 1 handful of fresh spinach
- 2 tbsp chopped walnuts
- 1 cup unsweetened almond milk (or your preferred milk)

Instructions:

1. Add the blueberries, spinach, turmeric, black pepper, and walnuts to a blender.
2. Pour in the almond milk.
3. Blend on high speed until smooth.
4. Pour into a glass and enjoy immediately.

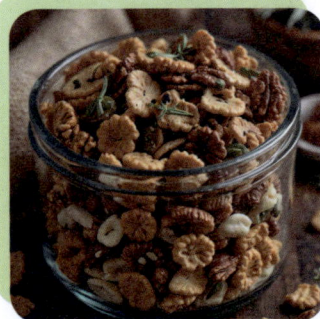

Crispy Rosemary & Walnuts Snack Mix

This snack mix combines rosemary for memory enhancement, walnuts for omega-3 fatty acids essential for cognitive health, and pumpkin seeds rich in zinc and magnesium to support memory retention.

Ingredients:

- 1 cup raw walnuts
- 1/2 cup pumpkin seeds
- 1 tsp dried rosemary
- 1 tbsp olive oil
- Sea salt to taste

Instructions:

1. Preheat the oven to 350°F (175°C).
2. In a bowl, mix the walnuts and pumpkin seeds with olive oil and rosemary.
3. Spread the mixture evenly on a baking sheet and sprinkle with sea salt.
4. Bake for 8-10 minutes or until golden and aromatic.
5. Let cool and enjoy as a brain-boosting snack.

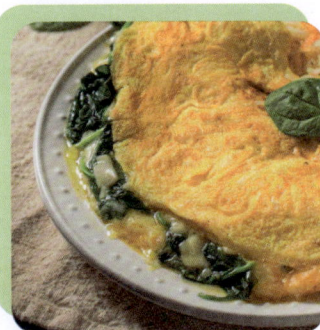

Lion's Mane & Spinach Brain Omelet

This omelet features lion's mane mushroom for neuroprotection, spinach for brain-supporting antioxidants and vitamins, and eggs rich in choline, essential for neurotransmitter production and memory function.

Ingredients:

- 2 eggs
- 1/2 cup chopped lion's mane mushroom
- 1/2 cup fresh spinach
- 1/4 tsp turmeric powder
- Salt and pepper to taste
- 1 tbsp olive oil or butter

Instructions:

1. Heat the olive oil or butter in a non-stick pan over medium heat.
2. Add the chopped lion's mane mushroom and sauté for 2-3 minutes.
3. Add the spinach and cook until wilted.
4. Whisk the eggs with turmeric, salt, and pepper, then pour over the mushroom and spinach mixture.
5. Cook until the eggs are set, folding the omelet in half. Serve hot.

Focus & Concentration

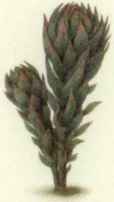

Rhodiola Rosea

Rhodiola is an adaptogenic herb that reduces mental fatigue and improves focus. Studies show it enhances cognitive performance and supports mental stamina under stress.

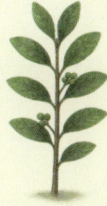

Yerba Mate

Yerba mate combines caffeine, theobromine, and antioxidants to enhance alertness and focus without the jittery effects of coffee. It boosts cognitive function, energy levels, and mental endurance.

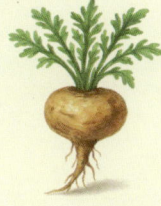

Maca Root

Maca is traditionally used to support energy and focus. Clinical studies suggest regular use can improve mental clarity, concentration, and overall cognitive performance.

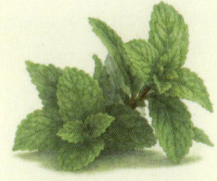

Peppermint

Peppermint improves focus and mental clarity through its stimulating aroma and menthol content. It enhances alertness, memory, oxygen flow, cognitive brain function, and overall mental performance.

Yerba Mate Energy Smoothie

This smoothie harnesses the natural caffeine and theobromine from yerba mate, combined with the healthy fats from avocado and antioxidants from spinach, to enhance concentration and mental stamina without the jitters.

Ingredients:

- 1 cup brewed and cooled yerba mate tea
- 1/2 ripe avocado
- 1 cup fresh spinach
- 1 tbsp honey or maple syrup (optional)
- Ice cubes (optional)

Instructions:

1. Add the brewed yerba mate, avocado, spinach, and honey (if using) to a blender.
2. Blend until smooth and creamy.
3. Add ice cubes for a chilled version.
4. Serve immediately for a refreshing and focus-enhancing treat.

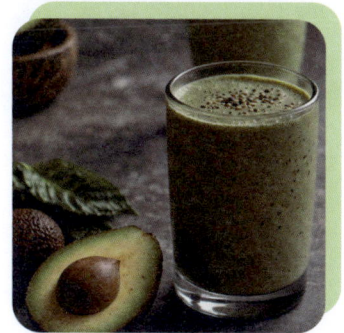

Bacopa & Dark Chocolate Energy Bites

Bacopa monnieri is a revered herb in Ayurvedic medicine for enhancing memory, reducing anxiety, and improving attention. When paired with antioxidant-rich dark chocolate and omega-3-rich walnuts, these bites make a potent snack for productivity and stress resilience.

Ingredients:

- 1 cup rolled oats
- 1–2 tsp Bacopa monnieri powder*
- ½ cup chopped walnuts
- ½ cup melted dark chocolate (70% cocoa or higher)
- 2 tbsp honey (or maple syrup for vegan option)

Instructions:

1. In a medium bowl, combine oats, bacopa powder, and chopped walnuts.
2. Pour in the melted dark chocolate and honey.
3. Mix thoroughly until all ingredients are evenly coated.
4. Roll the mixture into small, bite-sized balls using your hands or a cookie scoop.

*Start with 1 tsp if new to Bacopa's earthy taste, and adjust as tolerated.

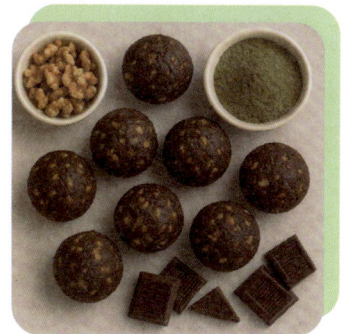

Rhodiola & Peppermint Iced Elixir

This iced elixir is designed to refresh and invigorate. The adaptogenic properties of rhodiola combined with peppermint's natural cognitive-boosting qualities create a potent drink to enhance focus during intense mental tasks.

Ingredients:

- 1 tsp dried rhodiola root (or 1 capsule content)
- 1 tsp dried peppermint leaves
- 1 tbsp lemon juice
- 1 tsp honey or agave syrup
- Ice cubes

Instructions:

1. Boil 1 cup of water and steep the rhodiola and peppermint for 10 minutes.
2. Strain the tea and let it cool.
3. Stir in lemon juice and honey, then pour over ice cubes.
4. Enjoy this iced drink during midday slumps to restore focus and concentration.

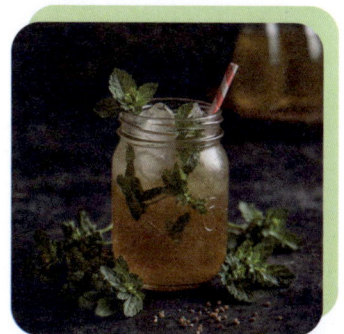

Anxiety & Stress Relief

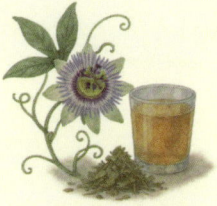

Passionflower

Passionflower is a natural anxiolytic that reduces anxiety without causing drowsiness. It boosts GABA levels in the brain, promoting calmness, as confirmed by clinical studies.

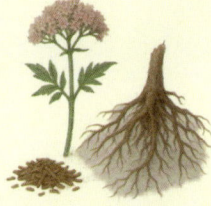

Valerian Root

Valerian root is well-known for calming effects and sleep support. Studies show it reduces anxiety and improves sleep quality, both important for managing stress.

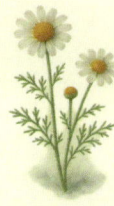

Chamomile

Chamomile contains apigenin, an antioxidant that binds to brain receptors to ease anxiety and promote relaxation. Research supports its use for mild to moderate anxiety.

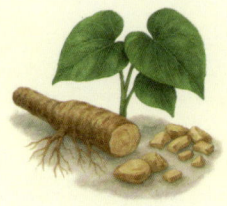

Kava

Kava, native to the Pacific Islands, is used traditionally for its calming effects. Kavalactones in kava interact with neurotransmitters to reduce anxiety and support relaxation.

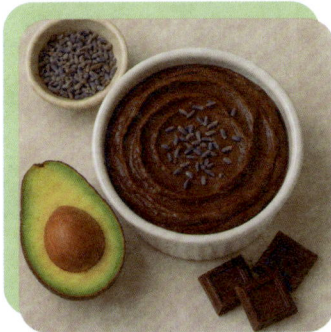

Dark Chocolate Avocado Mousse with Lavender

This mousse supports relaxation and mood through healthy fats from avocado, mood-enhancing antioxidants in dark chocolate, and calming effects of lavender, which helps reduce anxiety and promote restful sleep.

Ingredients:

- 1 ripe avocado
- ½ cup dark chocolate (70%+ cocoa)
- 2–3 tbsp milk (any kind)
- 1–2 tsp honey or maple syrup
- ½ tsp dried culinary grade lavender buds
- ½ tsp vanilla extract
- Pinch of sea salt

Instructions:

1. Warm milk with lavender over low heat for 3–5 mins (don't boil). Strain out lavender.
2. Melt chocolate in a double boiler or microwave in 20-sec bursts, stirring until smooth.
3. Blend avocado, melted chocolate, lavender milk, vanilla, sweetener, and salt until creamy.
4. Spoon into ramekins and chill for at least 1 hour.
5. Optional: Top with crushed walnuts, cacao nibs, yogurt, or a sprinkle of lavender.

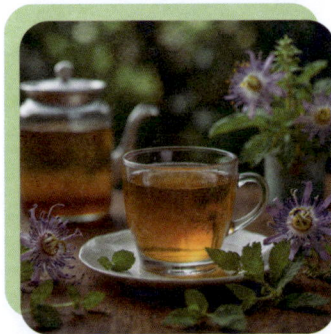

Stress-Relief Passionflower & Lemon Balm Tea

This tea combines the powerful anxiolytic effects of passionflower and lemon balm, enhanced with a touch of peppermint for a refreshing finish. It's designed to relax the body and mind while uplifting your spirits.

Ingredients:

- 1 tsp dried passionflower
- 1 tsp dried lemon balm
- 1/2 tsp dried peppermint
- 1 tsp honey (optional)

Instructions:

1. Combine the passionflower, lemon balm, and peppermint in a teapot.
2. Pour 1 cup of boiling water over the herbs and steep for 5-7 minutes.
3. Strain the tea, add honey if desired, and sip slowly to ease anxiety and stress.

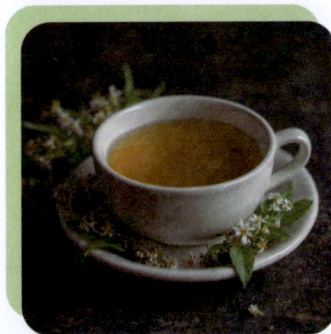

Valerian & Holy Basil Bedtime Elixir

This soothing elixir blends valerian root and holy basil, both known for their stress-relief and calming properties. This combination is ideal for promoting relaxation and preparing for restful sleep.

Ingredients:

- 1/2 tsp valerian root (dried)
- 1 tsp holy basil leaves (dried or fresh)
- 1/2 tsp chamomile flowers
- 1/2 cup warm coconut milk
- 1/2 tsp vanilla extract (optional for flavor)

Instructions:

1. Steep valerian root, holy basil, and chamomile
2. flowers in 1 cup of hot water for 5-7 minutes, then strain.
3. Warm the coconut milk and add it to the strained tea.
4. Add the vanilla extract for a comforting flavor.
5. Drink warm about an hour before bedtime to promote relaxation and alleviate stress.

Mood Balance

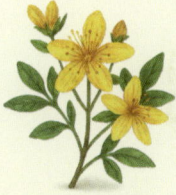

St. John's Wort

St. John's Wort is well-studied for mood regulation and is commonly used as a natural remedy for depression. Clinical trials show it boosts serotonin and may match antidepressants for mild cases.

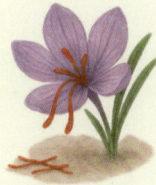

Saffron

Saffron has mood-lifting effects backed by multiple studies. Compounds like crocin and safranal help raise serotonin levels, improving mood and easing depressive symptoms.

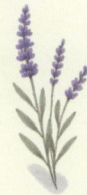

Lavender

Lavender, often used as tea or essential oil, is known for its calming and mood-balancing effects. Studies show it reduces anxiety, improves sleep, and supports emotional well-being.

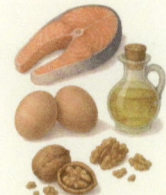

Omega-3 Fatty Acids

Omega-3 fatty acids are essential for brain health and emotional balance. Research links them to improved mood and reduced symptoms of depression and mental fatigue.

Tuna & Avocado Sushi Rolls

This sushi roll combines tuna and avocado—two nutrient-dense ingredients known to support mood balance and cognitive function. Tuna is a rich source of omega-3 fatty acids, and avocado adds creamy texture and is packed with magnesium and healthy monounsaturated fats.

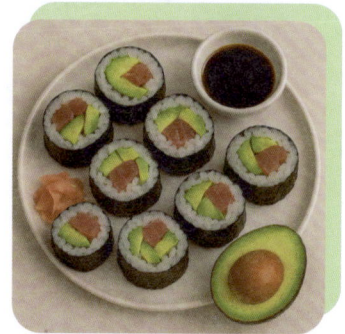

Ingredients:
- 1 cup cooked sushi rice
- 2 nori sheets
- ½ avocado, thinly sliced
- 100 g (3.5 oz) sushi-grade tuna (raw or cooked), sliced
- 1 tsp rice vinegar
- ¼ tsp sea salt
- Optional: sesame seeds, cucumber, tamari/soy sauce

Instructions:
1. Mix rice with vinegar and salt. Let cool.
2. Place nori (shiny side down) on a mat or towel.
3. Press ½ cup rice onto nori, leaving a 1-inch top border.
4. Add avocado, tuna, and optional cucumber across the bottom third.
5. Roll tightly from the bottom, sealing the edge with water.
6. Slice into 6–8 pieces with a wet knife. Top with sesame seeds or serve with tamari and ginger.

St. John's Wort Herbal Tea Blend

This calming herbal tea combines St. John's Wort, lemon balm, and lavender for a soothing, mood-balancing effect. St. John's Wort is known for its antidepressant properties, while lemon balm and lavender promote relaxation and emotional balance.

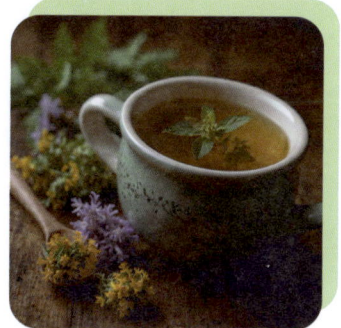

Ingredients:
- 1 tbsp dried St. John's Wort
- 1 tbsp dried lemon balm
- 1 tsp dried lavender flowers
- 2 cups boiling water
- Honey or lemon (optional)

Instructions:
1. Place all herbs in a teapot or infuser.
2. Pour the boiling water over the herbs and let steep for 5-7 minutes.
3. Strain and sweeten with honey or a squeeze of lemon if desired. Sip slowly to enhance relaxation.

Saffron & Holy Basil Golden Milk

This soothing drink blends saffron, holy basil, and turmeric to calm the mind and boost mood. Saffron and turmeric enhance serotonin, while holy basil reduces stress and balances cortisol.

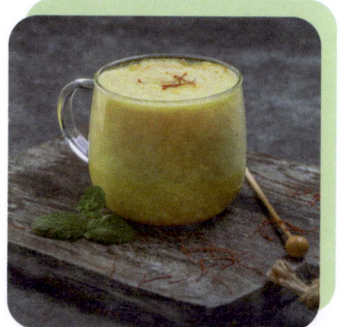

Ingredients:
- 1 cup warm milk (dairy or plant-based)
- 1/2 tsp turmeric powder
- 1/2 tsp saffron threads (steeped in 2 tbsp warm water)
- 1/2 tsp holy basil powder or 1 tsp holy basil extract
- 1 tsp honey or maple syrup for sweetness

Instructions:
1. Warm the milk in a saucepan over medium heat.
2. Add the turmeric, steeped saffron water, and holy basil to the milk, stirring until combined.
3. Sweeten with honey or maple syrup if desired.
4. Pour into a mug and enjoy before bedtime for a mood-balancing, stress-relieving ritual.

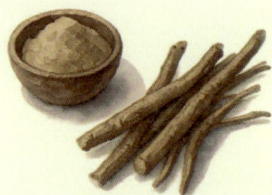

Sleep

Ashwagandha

Ashwagandha contains compounds like triethylene glycol that have sedative effects, reducing cortisol levels and promoting relaxation. This powerful adaptogenic herb helps balance the body's stress response, improving sleep quality, duration, and overall nighttime recovery.

- Take 300–500 mg of ashwagandha extract or ¼–½ teaspoon of powder in warm milk or water in the evening.

- 600 mg of ashwagandha extract daily for 8 weeks enhanced sleep quality by 72% in those with insomnia.[25]

- Pair ashwagandha with warm milk— milk's tryptophan enhances its calming power.

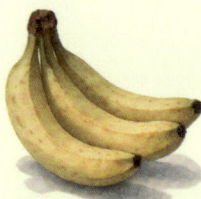

Bananas

Bananas are rich in potassium and magnesium, which relax muscles and calm the nervous system. They also contain tryptophan, an amino acid the body converts into melatonin and serotonin, supporting better sleep, balanced mood, and healthy sleep-wake cycles.

- Eat one banana about an hour before bed to promote natural relaxation.

- A banana before bed offers 32 mg of magnesium and 450 mg of potassium, which may aid relaxation and sleep.[26]

- For a sleep-boosting smoothie, blend a banana with a small handful of almonds and warm milk before bedtime.

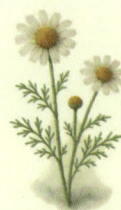

Chamomile

Chamomile contains apigenin, an antioxidant that binds to receptors in the brain, promoting relaxation and reducing anxiety, making it easier to fall asleep. Chamomile has mild sedative properties that have been used for centuries as a natural sleep aid.

- Drink one cup of chamomile tea 30 minutes before bed. Steep for at least 10 minutes for maximum effect.

- Chamomile tea can enhance sleep quality, lowering the Pittsburgh Sleep Quality Index score by 1.88 points.[27]

- Add a teaspoon of honey to chamomile tea, as the natural sugars help release serotonin, further promoting relaxation.

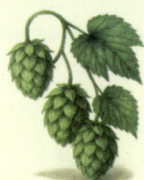

Hops

Known for its use in brewing, hops also have natural sedative properties due to their active compound, methylbutenol. This compound calms the central nervous system, relieving anxiety and promoting drowsiness without impairing next-day alertness or causing habit-forming side effects.

- Consume 0.5 -1 g of dried hops in tea or take 100 mg of hops extract 1–2 hours before bed.

- Drinking non-alcoholic beer with hops at dinner enhanced sleep quality by 7% in university students.[28]

- Hops pair well with chamomile or valerian in teas, enhancing its calming effect and helping you drift off faster.

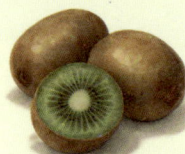

Kiwis

Kiwis are packed with antioxidants, including serotonin-producing compounds, which help regulate sleep and mood naturally and effectively. They also contain folate, which may reduce insomnia symptoms, and fiber, which supports steady blood sugar, healthy digestion, and restful sleep throughout the night.

- Eat two kiwis one hour before bedtime for best results.

- Two kiwifruits an hour before bed for four weeks helped adults fall asleep 35% faster and sleep 13% longer.[29]

- Kiwis and almonds make a sleep-boosting snack packed with melatonin, magnesium, and serotonin-supporting nutrients.

Lavender

Lavender contains linalool and linalyl acetate, compounds with calming effects on the nervous system that help reduce stress, anxiety, and nervous tension. It interacts with GABA receptors, promoting relaxation, easing tension, and aiding in faster sleep onset, deeper rest, and better sleep quality overall.

- Use 1–2 drops of lavender oil in a diffuser before bed, or brew lavender tea with 1–2 tsp of dried flowers.

- Smelling lavender oil before bed enhances sleep quality by 2.5 points on the Pittsburgh Sleep Quality Index.[30]

- Place dried lavender by your pillow or apply diluted oil to pulse points for all-night relaxation.

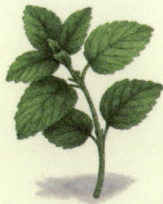

Lemon Balm

Lemon balm, a member of the mint family, contains rosmarinic acid, which boosts GABA levels in the brain. This helps ease anxiety, calm the mind, and improve sleep quality by reducing nighttime awakenings, restlessness, and promoting deeper, more restorative sleep.

Brew 1–2 teaspoons of dried lemon balm for 10 minutes, or take as a tincture (30–40 drops in water).

Consuming 600 mg of lemon balm extract daily for 15 days decreased insomnia symptoms by 42%.[31]

Combine lemon balm with valerian root tea for a stronger, synergistic effect to support deeper relaxation and sleep.

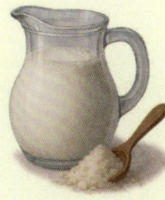

Milk (Warm Milk)

Warm milk contains tryptophan, an amino acid that promotes serotonin production. This is then converted to melatonin, which regulates sleep cycles. Drinking warm milk before bed can have a calming effect, reduce stress, and support a healthy sleep routine.

Drink 1 cup of warm milk 20–30 minutes before bed; add nutmeg or cinnamon to boost its calming effects.

One study found that drinking warm milk with honey before bed for three days improved sleep quality by 14%.[32]

Choose unsweetened organic milk and pair it with a light carbohydrate snack, like toast, to boost tryptophan absorption.

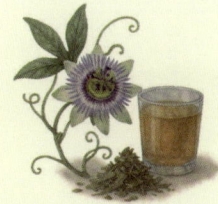

Passionflower

Passionflower boosts GABA levels in the brain, helping calm the mind, ease anxiety, and improve sleep quality and duration naturally and effectively. It's especially effective for people whose sleep problems are caused by stress, nervous tension, or overactive thoughts at night.

Brew 1 teaspoon of passionflower for 10 minutes before bed, or take 250–500 mg of extract an hour before.

Drinking passionflower tea each night for a week enhanced sleep quality by 5% in healthy adults.[33]

Pair passionflower with chamomile or lemon balm for a stronger calming tea. Avoid high doses to prevent daytime drowsiness.

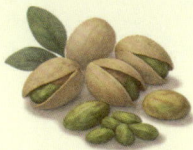

Pistachios

Pistachios contain melatonin, a hormone that helps regulate sleep-wake cycles, along with magnesium and vitamin B6, which help produce serotonin and melatonin, encouraging better sleep quality, deeper rest, reduced nighttime awakenings, enhanced relaxation, and overall improved nighttime recovery and wellness.

Eat a small handful (20–30 g) of pistachios in the evening, or add to yogurt or salad before bed.

A 100 g serving of pistachios contains about 23 mg of melatonin, much more than most foods or supplements.[34]

Keep shelled pistachios by your bedside – eating a few 1–2 hours before sleep may gently raise melatonin and help you drift off.

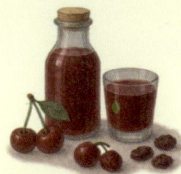

Tart Cherry Juice

Tart cherries are naturally high in melatonin, the hormone that regulates the sleep-wake cycle. Drinking tart cherry juice may increase melatonin levels in the body, improving sleep quality, duration, and recovery, while reducing insomnia symptoms and nighttime awakenings in a safe, natural way without next-day grogginess or dependence.

Drink 8 oz of tart cherry juice in the evening, about 1–2 hours before bed, for best results.

Drinking 240 mL of tart cherry juice twice daily for two weeks added 84 minutes of sleep in adults with insomnia.[35]

Opt for 100% pure tart cherry juice with no added sugars, as sugar may interfere with sleep quality.

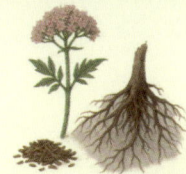

Valerian Root

Valerian root contains valerenic acid, which inhibits the breakdown of GABA, a calming neurotransmitter. This helps with relaxation, reduces anxiety, and improves sleep. It is particularly effective for reducing mild insomnia, sleep latency, nighttime restlessness, nervous tension, and enhancing overall sleep duration and quality.

Take 300–600 mg of valerian 30–60 minutes before bed, or brew 1 teaspoon of root for 10–15 minutes.

Taking valerian root can enhance sleep quality by 1.8 times compared to a placebo.[36]

Combine valerian with lemon balm or passionflower for added calm. Start with a low dose to assess effects.

Insomnia & Sleep Disorders

EXTRA HERBS

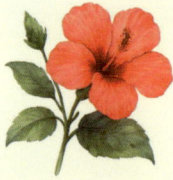

Hibiscus

Hibiscus is rich in antioxidants and vitamin C, traditionally used for its calming effects. It helps support balanced blood pressure, easing tension and promoting restful sleep.

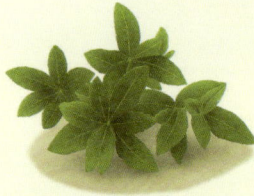

Lemon Verbena

Lemon verbena is known for its relaxing properties. It contains verbascoside, a compound with mild sedative effects that help reduce anxiety, calm the nervous system, and support deeper sleep.

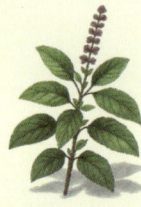

Holy Basil (Tulsi)

Holy Basil helps lower stress and cortisol levels, which can disrupt sleep. Studies show it promotes relaxation and improves sleep quality, especially in stress-related insomnia.

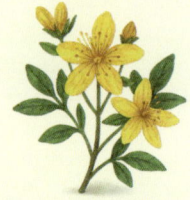

St. John's Wort

St. John's Wort contains hypericin, which influences serotonin levels. It supports mood and can help relieve insomnia, particularly when linked to anxiety or mild depression.

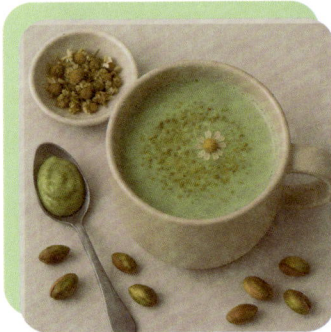

Dreamy Pistachio & Chamomile Milk

This soothing blend pairs calming chamomile with melatonin-rich pistachios and warm milk to promote restful sleep. Chamomile eases anxiety, while pistachios provide magnesium and B6 to support serotonin and nervous system balance.

Ingredients:

- 1 cup warm milk (dairy or unsweetened plant milk)
- 1 tbsp pistachio butter (or 2 tbsp finely ground pistachios)
- 1 chamomile tea bag (or 1 tsp dried chamomile flowers)
- 1 tsp honey (optional, for sweetness)

Instructions:

1. Warm the milk gently on the stove, making sure not to boil it.
2. Add the chamomile tea bag to the milk and let it steep for 5–7 minutes.
3. Remove the tea bag, then stir in the pistachio butter or ground pistachios and add honey if using.
4. Sip slowly about 30 minutes before bed to support relaxation and deep sleep.

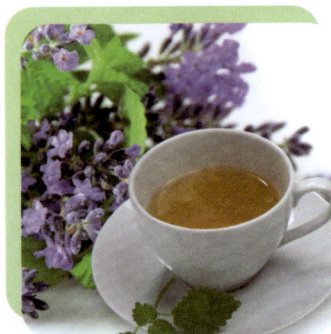

Lavender & Lemon Balm Sleep Tonic

This calming tonic combines lavender and lemon balm to reduce anxiety and enhance sleep. Lavender provides sedative effects, while lemon balm decreases stress and improves sleep onset, promoting better sleep quality.

Ingredients:

- 1 tsp dried lavender flowers
- 1 tsp dried lemon balm
- 1 cup hot water
- 1 tsp tart cherry juice (optional, for flavor and melatonin boost)

Instructions:

1. Steep the lavender and lemon balm in hot water for 8-10 minutes.
2. Strain the herbs, adding a splash of tart cherry juice if desired for taste and extra sleep support.
3. Enjoy this tea 1 hour before bedtime to prepare for restful sleep.

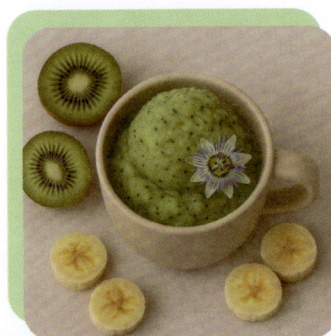

Kiwi, Banana & Passionflower Sorbet

This refreshing sorbet combines kiwi, banana, and passionflower—ingredients known to support better sleep. Kiwi and banana provide antioxidants, magnesium, and B6 to boost melatonin and serotonin. Passionflower helps calm the mind and ease restlessness, making it a perfect dessert for winding down.

Ingredients:

- 2 ripe kiwis, chopped
- 1 ripe banana, sliced
- ¼ cup cooled passionflower tea
- 1–2 tsp honey or maple syrup (optional)
- ½ tsp lemon juice (optional)

Instructions:

1. Freeze kiwi and banana for at least 4 hours.
2. Blend with cooled passionflower tea until smooth.
3. Add sweetener or lemon juice if needed; blend again.
4. Serve immediately (soft-serve) or freeze 1 hour for a firmer texture.

Sleep Quality & Recovery

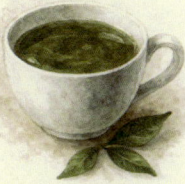

Green Tea

Green tea contains L-theanine, a calming compound that increases alpha brain waves, promoting relaxation and reducing stress. Decaffeinated green tea may help improve sleep quality.

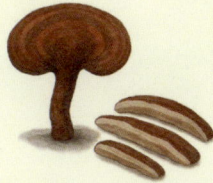

Reishi Mushroom

Reishi mushrooms are rich in calming triterpenes that ease stress and enhance sleep quality. They also support immune health, promote relaxation, and aid in deeper recovery during rest.

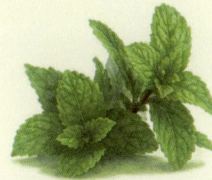

Peppermint

Peppermint relaxes muscles, soothes digestion, and eases breathing discomfort. It supports better sleep, especially for those experiencing disrupted rest due to tension or congestion.

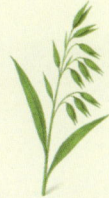

Oat Straw

Oat straw is high in calcium and magnesium, which help calm the nervous system. It promotes deep relaxation, supports restorative sleep, and reduces night-time disturbances, stress, and tension.

Soothing Almond-Banana Smoothie

This smoothie blends magnesium-rich almonds and potassium-packed bananas to relax muscles and promote restful sleep. Both contain tryptophan, supporting serotonin and melatonin production for better sleep quality.

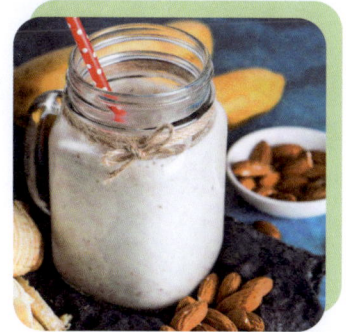

Ingredients:
- 1 banana
- 1 tbsp almond butter (or a handful of soaked almonds)
- 1 cup warm almond milk (or regular warm milk)
- 1 tsp honey (optional for added sweetness and soothing effect)

Instructions:
1. In a blender, combine the banana, almond butter, and warm almond milk.
2. Blend until smooth.
3. Pour into a glass and add honey if desired. Enjoy this warm, creamy smoothie about an
4. hour before bed to ease into relaxation.

Lavender Chamomile Bedtime Tea

This calming tea combines lavender and chamomile, both rich in compounds that calm the nervous system, reduce anxiety, and promote sleep quality. This herbal blend is ideal for unwinding at night, helping you drift into restorative sleep.

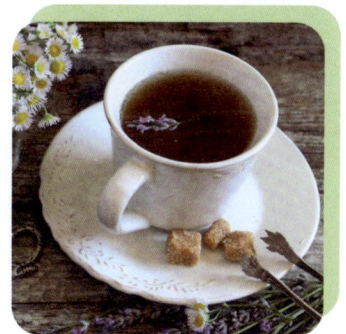

Ingredients:
- 1 tsp dried lavender
- 1 tsp chamomile
- 1 tsp lemon balm (optional)
- 1 cup hot water
- Honey to taste (optional)

Instructions:
1. Add the lavender, chamomile, and lemon balm to a tea infuser or teapot.
2. Pour hot water over the herbs and let steep for 5-7 minutes.
3. Strain the tea into a cup and add honey if desired.
4. Sip slowly, inhaling the soothing aroma to ease into relaxation.

Tart Cherry & Passionflower Sleep Tonic

Tart cherry juice is a natural source of melatonin, helping to regulate the sleep-wake cycle. Passionflower adds a calming effect, reducing restlessness and promoting a deeper sleep, making this tonic a potent aid for high-quality recovery sleep.

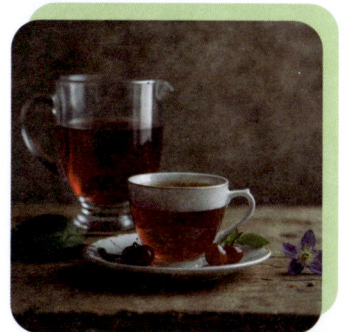

Ingredients:
- 1/2 cup tart cherry juice
- 1/2 cup warm water
- 1 tsp passionflower extract or 1 tea bag of passionflower tea
- 1/2 tsp honey (optional)

Instructions:
1. Warm tart cherry juice and water.
2. Add passionflower extract or steep tea bag for 5 mins.
3. Remove tea bag (if used) and stir in honey if desired.
4. Drink 30 mins before bed to support natural sleep.

Immune System

Strengthen your immunity naturally – discover herbs and foods that support a robust immune system, keeping you protected year-round.

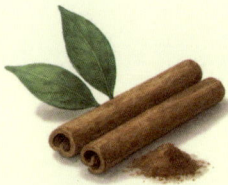

Cinnamon

Cinnamon contains cinnamaldehyde, a powerful compound with antimicrobial effects, helping to inhibit the growth of bacteria and fungi. Its antioxidant and anti-inflammatory properties also support immune resilience by reducing oxidative stress.

- Add 1/2 to 1 teaspoon of ground cinnamon to tea, smoothies, or meals daily.

- Cinnamon extract may reduce inflammation by inhibiting NF-κB activation by 50%.[37]

- Use Ceylon cinnamon for higher antioxidant benefits and less coumarin, a compound that can be harsh in large amounts.

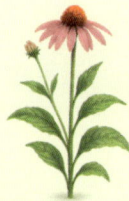

Echinacea

Echinacea is known for its ability to increase white blood cell production, which helps the body fight infections. The herb contains compounds that enhance immune activity, reduce inflammation, and increase resilience, making it particularly effective in shortening cold and flu symptoms.

- Take 1-2 g of dried echinacea root daily, or add to tea.

- Taking Echinacea may lower the chance of recurrent respiratory infections by 35%.[38]

- Use echinacea root instead of leaves for a stronger immune-boosting effect and greater therapeutic benefits.

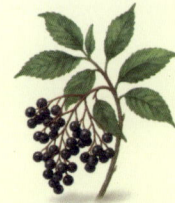

Elderberry

Elderberry is rich in flavonoids, especially anthocyanins, which give it potent antiviral properties. It inhibits viral replication, making it effective in reducing the duration of colds and flu. Elderberry also boosts cytokine production, enhancing immune response.

- Take 1 tablespoon of elderberry syrup daily, or increase to 1 tablespoon every few hours during illness.

- Taking elderberry supplements might shorten flu symptoms by about 2 days.[39]

- Pair elderberry with honey for added antiviral benefits and to soothe a sore throat, reduce coughing, and support faster recovery.

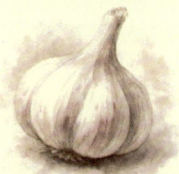

Garlic

Garlic's active compound, allicin, has potent antimicrobial and antiviral effects that help combat infections and support immune health. It also boosts the activity of immune cells, such as natural killer cells, which defend the body against viruses and other harmful pathogens while reducing inflammation and oxidative stress.

- Consume 1-2 raw cloves daily, or add 1 teaspoon minced garlic to meals.

- Taking aged garlic extract daily may decrease the occurrence of the common cold by 61%.[40]

- Crush or chop garlic and let it sit for 10 minutes before use to maximize allicin production, boosting its antimicrobial and immune-strengthening effects.

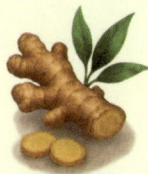

Ginger

Ginger contains gingerol, a bioactive compound with powerful anti-inflammatory and antimicrobial properties. It helps relieve respiratory infections, soothes sore throats, and strengthens the immune system. Its natural warming effect also enhances circulation, supporting immunity and promoting faster recovery.

- Grate 1-2 teaspoons of fresh ginger into tea or meals daily.

- Taking 20 mg of gingerols daily may ease inflammation in autoimmune conditions by calming the immune response.[41]

- For stronger effects, pair ginger with honey and lemon in a warm tea, as these ingredients create a powerful immune-boosting synergy.

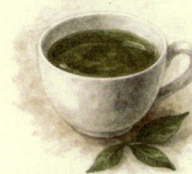

Green Tea

Green tea is rich in catechins, especially EGCG, which have powerful antiviral and immune-boosting effects. These compounds help fight pathogens, reduce inflammation, and support immune cell function, helping prevent infections like the flu and enhancing overall immune resilience.

- Aim for 1-3 cups of green tea daily.

- Drinking six cups of green tea daily may strengthen your immune defenses by boosting key immune cells.[42]

- Add lemon to green tea to boost catechin absorption by up to 80%, for good immune support, antioxidant activity, and overall health benefits.

Immune System

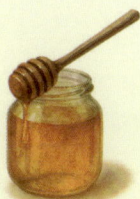

Honey

Honey contains enzymes and natural compounds that boost the immune response and fight infection. Its antimicrobial properties help reduce sore throat symptoms and support wound healing. High antioxidant content makes it beneficial in combating oxidative stress.

Take 1-2 teaspoon daily, especially raw or manuka honey for enhanced effects.

Consuming 70 g of honey daily for a month may boost antioxidant defenses.[43]

Add a teaspoon of honey to warm lemon water in the morning for a daily immune boost, improved digestion, and natural hydration.

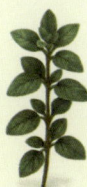

Oregano

Oregano contains carvacrol and thymol, powerful compounds with strong antimicrobial effects that help fight off bacteria and fungi. Its potent antioxidants further support immune health by reducing oxidative stress, enhancing defenses, and protecting cells from damage.

Use 1-2 drops of oregano oil in water (diluted) or 1 teaspoon of fresh oregano in meals.

Carvacrol in oregano oil may boost HSP70 levels, potentially reducing autoimmune arthritis symptoms.[44]

Use dried oregano in soups and broths to release its immune-boosting oils, enhance flavor, and support respiratory health.

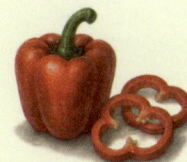

Red Bell Pepper

Red bell peppers are packed with vitamin C and antioxidants like beta-carotene. Vitamin C boosts immune cell function, supports white blood cell production, and acts as a powerful antioxidant, helping the immune system fight infection and reduce inflammation.

Eat raw or cooked red peppers daily. Even ½ cup of raw red pepper provides ~95 mg of vitamin C.

Red bell pepper leaf extract helps support the immune system by reducing inflammation without harming cells.[45]

Keep sliced red pepper sticks in the fridge for an easy snack. They're crunchy, sweet, and deliver a big immunity boost.

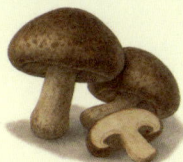

Shiitake Mushrooms

Shiitake mushrooms are high in beta-glucans, which enhance the activity of white blood cells, strengthening the body's immune defense system. They also provide essential minerals and vitamins that support immune health, reduce inflammation, fight infections, boost vitality, and promote overall wellness.

Add 1/4 cup of cooked shiitake mushrooms to meals 2-3 times weekly.

5–10 grams of shiitake mushrooms daily for a month may raise key immune cell activity by 60% and 30%.[46]

Sun-dry shiitake mushrooms before cooking to increase their vitamin D content, support bone health, and enhance immune function.

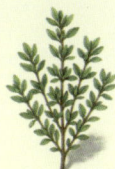

Thyme

Thyme contains thymol, a powerful polyphenolic compound with antibacterial and antiviral properties, making it especially effective against respiratory infections. Its potent antioxidant capacity helps protect cells from damage, reduce overall inflammation, and strengthen the immune system naturally.

Steep 1-2 teaspoons of thyme leaves in hot water for a daily immune tea.

Thyme essential oil may help regulate immune responses by decreasing IL-6 levels by 75% and TNF-α levels by 40%.[47]

Inhale steam from thyme-infused hot water to relieve congestion, soothe airways, and support respiratory health.

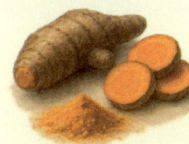

Turmeric

Turmeric's active compound, curcumin, reduces inflammation and boosts immune response by enhancing antibody production and modulating immune cell activity. It's especially helpful in managing chronic inflammation, supporting detoxification, and promoting overall immune balance and resilience.

Take 1/2 teaspoon of turmeric daily, ideally with a pinch of black pepper for absorption.

Adding turmeric to your diet may lower inflammatory markers by up to 50%, supporting immune balance.[48]

Combine with honey and ginger in warm water for a potent anti-inflammatory tonic for immunity boost.

Immune Boosting Herbs

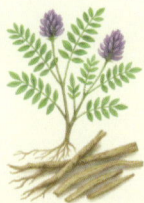

Astragalus

Astragalus is rich in immune-boosting polysaccharides. It enhances white blood cell activity and strengthens resistance to infections, especially during seasonal changes.

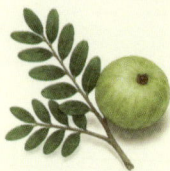

Amla (Indian Gooseberry)

Amla is high in vitamin C and antioxidants. It boosts immunity, fights pathogens, and supports immune function through its antibacterial and anti-inflammatory properties.

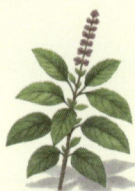

Holy Basil (Tulsi)

Holy Basil supports immune health by reducing inflammation and stress, two key factors that weaken immunity. It also enhances respiratory defense, balances cortisol levels, and strengthens immune response.

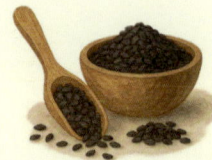

Black Cumin Seed

Black cumin seed is rich in thymoquinone, which boosts immune cell activity and reduces inflammation. It's traditionally used to strengthen immunity and fight infections.

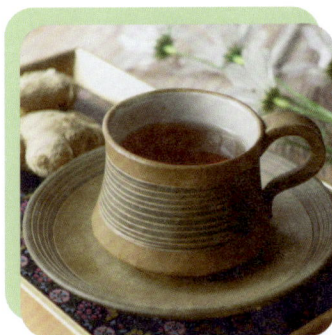

Cinnamon Ginger Immunity Elixir

Cinnamon and ginger's antioxidant and anti-inflammatory benefits boost immunity. Combined with lemon and honey, they form a warming elixir to strengthen defenses and prevent infections.

Ingredients:
- 1 cup of hot water
- 1/2 tsp ground cinnamon
- 1/2 tsp grated fresh ginger (or 1/4 teaspoon ground ginger)
- Juice of 1/2 lemon
- 1 tbsp honey

Instructions:
1. Add cinnamon and grated ginger to the hot water.
2. Let steep for 5 minutes, then add the lemon juice and honey, stirring well.
3. Sip slowly and enjoy warm, preferably in the morning or evening to maximize immune support.

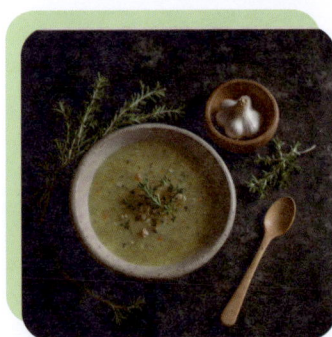

Thyme & Garlic Immunity Soup

Garlic and thyme, with their antimicrobial properties, are powerful immune boosters. This simple soup strengthens defenses, especially during cold and flu season.

Ingredients:
- 2 cups vegetable or chicken broth
- 3 cloves garlic, minced
- 1/2 tsp dried thyme (or 1 tsp fresh thyme, chopped)
- 1/4 tsp turmeric powder
- Salt and pepper to taste

Instructions:
1. Simmer broth in a small pot over medium heat.
2. Add garlic, thyme, and turmeric.
3. Simmer 5–10 mins to blend flavors.
4. Season with salt and pepper. Enjoy warm.

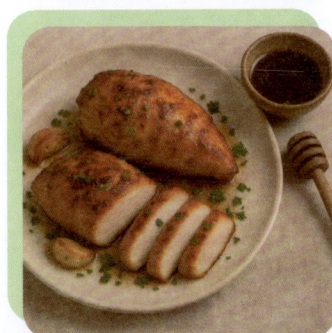

Honey & Garlic Chicken

This dish pairs garlic's immune-boosting power with honey's soothing, antibacterial properties. Chicken adds protein to support healing and immune cell function, making it a nourishing meal for daily immune support.

Ingredients (Serves 2–3):
- 2–3 boneless chicken breasts or thighs
- 4 garlic cloves, minced
- 2 tbsp raw honey
- 1 tbsp olive oil
- 1 tbsp soy sauce or tamari
- 1 tbsp lemon juice or ACV
- ½ tsp dried thyme
- Salt & pepper to taste
- Fresh parsley or green onion (garnish)

Instructions:
1. Mix garlic, honey, olive oil, soy sauce, lemon juice, and thyme into a marinade.
2. Season the chicken and marinate it for at least 30 minutes.
3. Cook the chicken in a skillet for 5–6 minutes per side until fully cooked.
4. Simmer leftover marinade for 2–3 minutes to thicken.
5. Drizzle sauce over chicken, garnish, and serve.

Cold & Flu Prevention

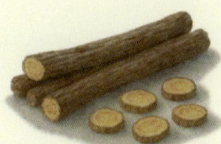

Licorice Root

Licorice root contains glycyrrhizin, which has antiviral effects effective against respiratory infections. It also soothes the throat and reduces inflammation, aiding cold and flu prevention.

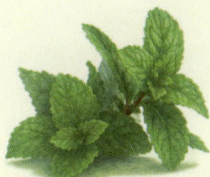

Peppermint

Peppermint is rich in menthol, which eases congestion and throat discomfort. It has antiviral and anti-inflammatory properties that relieve cold and flu symptoms and support respiratory health.

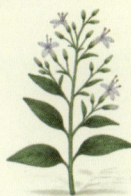

Andrographis

Andrographis is known for its antiviral and immune-boosting benefits. Studies show it helps prevent and lessen the severity of upper respiratory infections during cold season.

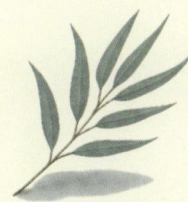

Eucalyptus

Eucalyptus has natural antiviral and anti-inflammatory properties. Inhalation of its oil opens airways and may reduce infection spread, helping with both prevention and symptom relief.

Turmeric Hummus with Bell Pepper Sticks

This recipe blends turmeric's anti-inflammatory curcumin with vitamin C–rich bell peppers to support immune function. Together, they help reduce oxidative stress and boost immune cell production.

Ingredients:

- 1 can (400 g) chickpeas, rinsed
- 2 tbsp tahini
- 1 tbsp lemon juice
- 1 tbsp olive oil
- 1 garlic clove, minced
- ½ tsp turmeric
- ¼ tsp cumin (optional)
- Salt & pepper to taste
- 2–4 tbsp cold water (as needed)
- Pinch of black pepper

For dipping:

- 2–3 bell peppers (red or yellow), sliced into sticks

Instructions:

1. Combine all ingredients in a food processor.
2. Blend until smooth, adding water as needed.
3. Adjust seasoning to taste.
4. Transfer to a bowl, drizzle with olive oil, and sprinkle turmeric or paprika (optional).
5. Serve with bell pepper sticks.

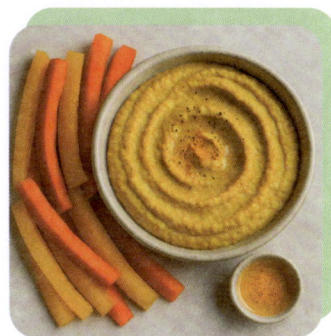

Immune-Boosting Turmeric & Green Tea Tonic

This tonic combines turmeric's anti-inflammatory benefits with green tea's antioxidants to boost immunity and protect against oxidative stress during cold and flu season.

Ingredients:

- 1 green tea bag
- 1/2 tsp turmeric powder
- 1 tsp honey
- Juice of 1/2 lemon
- 1 cup hot water

Instructions:

1. Place the green tea bag in a cup, add hot water, and let it steep for 3-5 minutes.
2. Remove the tea bag, then add turmeric powder and stir well.
3. Add honey and lemon juice, stirring to combine.
4. Enjoy this warm, immune-boosting tonic once daily.

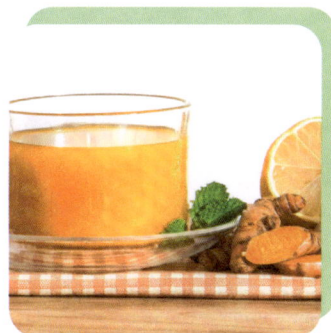

Cinnamon & Elderberry Syrup

Elderberry has been shown to reduce the severity and duration of colds and flu, while cinnamon provides warming and antimicrobial benefits. This syrup is easy to make, tastes delicious, and can be stored for regular preventive use.

Ingredients:

- 1/2 cup dried elderberries
- 1 cinnamon stick or 1 teaspoon cinnamon powder
- 1 cup water
- 1/4 cup raw honey

Instructions:

1. Simmer elderberries, cinnamon, and water for 15–20 mins until reduced by half.
2. Strain and let cool.
3. Stir in honey and store in the fridge.
4. Take 1–2 tsp daily, or 1 tbsp if symptoms arise.

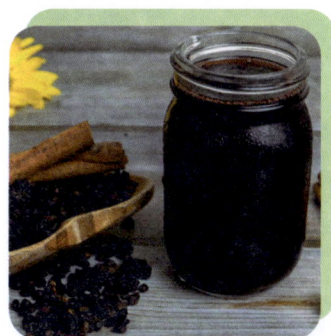

Autoimmune Support

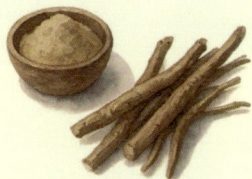

Astragalus

Astragalus is rich in immune-boosting polysaccharides. It enhances white blood cell activity and strengthens resistance to infections, especially during seasonal changes.

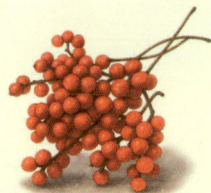

Schisandra Berry

Schisandra is an adaptogenic berry with powerful anti-inflammatory properties. It supports adrenal function and helps regulate immune activity, making it especially useful for autoimmune support.

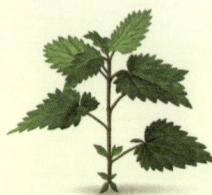

Stinging Nettle

Stinging nettle contains compounds that help regulate immune responses and lower inflammation. It's especially helpful for autoimmune issues affecting the joints, muscles, and connective tissues.

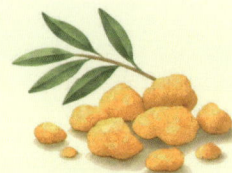

Boswellia

Boswellia supports autoimmune health by reducing inflammation and balancing immune responses, helping manage overactive immune activity without harsh side effects.

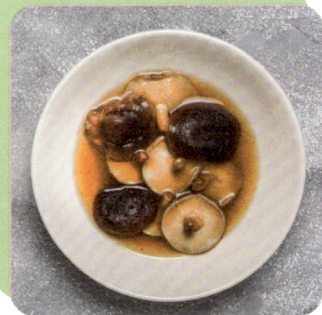

Shiitake Immune-Boosting Broth

Shiitake mushrooms contain beta-glucans, which help modulate immune responses, making this broth ideal for supporting autoimmune health. Combined with garlic and ginger, this broth helps reduce inflammation and promote balanced immune activity.

Ingredients:
- 4-5 dried or fresh shiitake mushrooms
- 2 cloves garlic, minced
- 1/2 inch fresh ginger, sliced
- 4 cups vegetable or chicken broth
- 1/4 tsp turmeric (optional)

Instructions:
1. In a pot, bring the broth to a boil.
2. Add the mushrooms, garlic, and ginger.
3. Simmer on low heat for 15-20 minutes.
4. Remove from heat, add turmeric if desired, and sip warm.

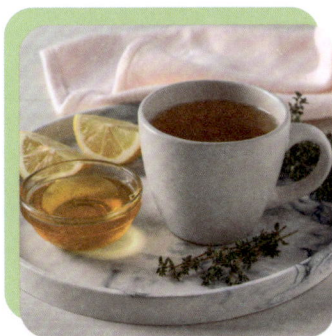

Lemon & Honey Immune Soother

This classic lemon and honey blend is enhanced with thyme, known for its antibacterial and anti-inflammatory properties, making it great for soothing autoimmune symptoms. Together, they support immune balance and help manage inflammatory responses.

Ingredients:
- Juice of 1 lemon
- 1 tsp raw honey
- 1/4 tsp dried thyme (or 1 sprig fresh thyme)
- 1 cup hot water

Instructions:
1. Add lemon juice and honey to a cup of hot water.
2. Stir in thyme and let it steep for 5 minutes.
3. Strain if desired, and enjoy warm.

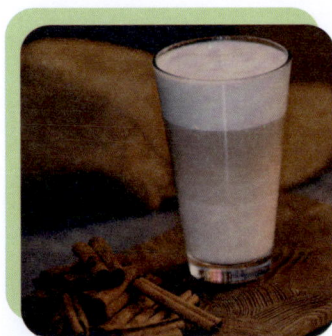

Cinnamon & Green Tea Immunity Latte

This comforting latte blends cinnamon and green tea to support immune health and reduce inflammation, ideal for autoimmune support. Antioxidants and immune-balancing properties make it both nourishing and delicious.

Ingredients:
- 1 cup brewed green tea
- 1/2 tsp ground cinnamon
- 1/2 tsp raw honey or maple syrup (optional)
- 1/4 cup almond milk (or milk of choice)

Instructions:
1. Brew green tea as usual and pour it into a mug.
2. Stir in cinnamon and honey or maple syrup if desired.
3. Add almond milk and enjoy warm for a soothing immunity boost.

Recovery Post Illness

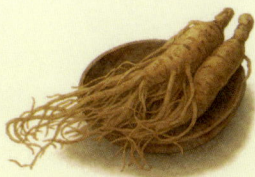

Ginseng (Panax)

Ginseng supports immune recovery by boosting energy, reducing fatigue, and enhancing immune function. It's well-studied for shortening recovery time and improving cellular immunity.

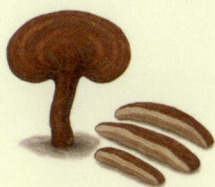

Reishi Mushroom

Reishi, known as the "mushroom of immortality," boosts immune cell activity and reduces fatigue. Its adaptogenic effects help balance immunity, reduce stress, and speed recovery after illness.

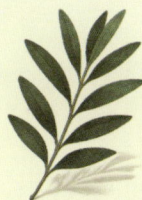

Olive Leaf

Olive leaf contains oleuropein, a potent antiviral and antimicrobial compound. It helps fight lingering infections and strengthens immunity during the recovery process.

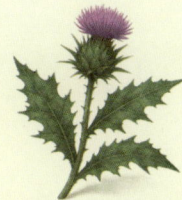

Milk Thistle

Milk thistle supports liver detoxification, a key part of recovery. Its antioxidant properties help clear toxins, restore energy, and improve immune resilience and overall vitality post-illness.

Honey Lemon Echinacea Tea

Echinacea is widely recognized for its immune-strengthening properties, especially during recovery. Combined with honey and lemon, this tea helps ease lingering fatigue and supports overall immune rejuvenation.

Ingredients:

- 1 cup hot water
- 1 echinacea tea bag or 1 teaspoon dried echinacea
- 1 tbsp honey
- Juice of half a lemon

Instructions:

1. Steep echinacea tea bag or dried echinacea in hot water for 5-7 minutes.
2. Stir in honey and lemon juice until well mixed.
3. Sip slowly while warm, 1-2 times a day to support post-illness recovery.

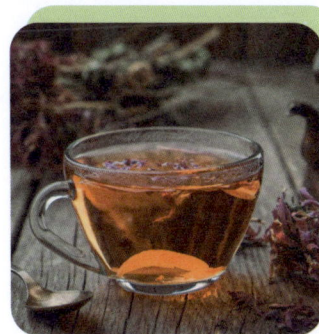

Garlic-Honey Immunity Elixir

Garlic and honey form a potent combination for immune recovery due to garlic's antimicrobial properties and honey's natural antioxidants. This simple elixir provides a gentle yet effective immune boost.

Ingredients:

- 1 garlic clove, finely minced
- 1 tbsp raw honey

Instructions:

1. Mix minced garlic with raw honey in a small bowl or jar.
2. Let it sit for 10 minutes to blend flavors.
3. Take this mixture once daily, either as-is or mixed with warm water, for a gentle immune lift.

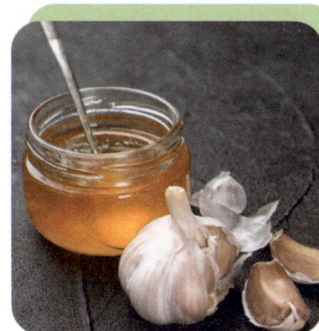

Cinnamon-Thyme Immune Support Tea

This warming tea combines cinnamon's antioxidant power with thyme's antimicrobial properties, creating a soothing drink to help the body recover strength and immunity after illness.

Ingredients:

- 1 cup hot water
- 1/2 tsp cinnamon powder or 1 cinnamon stick
- 1/2 tsp dried thyme
- 1 tsp honey (optional)

Instructions:

1. Add cinnamon and thyme to hot water.
2. Let steep for 5 minutes, then strain.
3. Stir in honey if desired and drink warm.
4. Enjoy once a day to support immune recovery naturally.

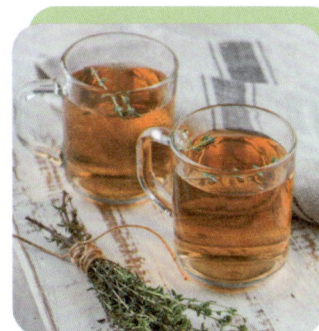

Respiratory Health

Breathe easier – learn about natural ways to support lung function, clear airways, and improve overall respiratory health.

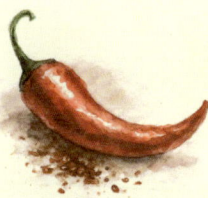

Cayenne Pepper

Cayenne pepper contains capsaicin, which helps thin mucus and relieve congestion. It also improves blood flow to the respiratory tract, aiding oxygen delivery and lung function. Capsaicin's warming effect opens up airways, providing relief for blocked sinuses.

Add 1/4 teaspoon of cayenne powder to warm water with lemon, drink once daily.

Capsaicin in cayenne pepper can enhance nasal airflow by 44% in non-allergic rhinitis sufferers.[49]

For added effect, mix with honey and ginger to soothe throat irritation, boost immunity, and enhance anti-inflammatory benefits.

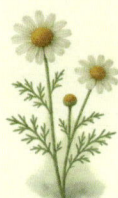

Chamomile

Chamomile's natural anti-inflammatory and antioxidant compounds calm irritated airways, reduce coughing, and ease sinus inflammation. Its mild sedative effect can help promote restful sleep, allowing the body to recover from respiratory distress faster.

Steep 1–2 teaspoons of chamomile flowers in hot water for 10 minutes; inhale steam and drink twice daily.

In a study of 154 patients with acute coronary syndrome, inhaling chamomile oil significantly lowered heart rate and blood pressure.[50]

Add a few drops of chamomile oil to hot water for an enhanced steam inhalation experience promoting relaxation.

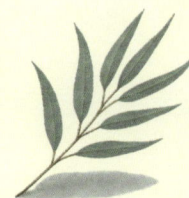

Eucalyptus

Eucalyptus contains eucalyptol, a compound that helps clear mucus and reduce airway inflammation. It also acts as an antimicrobial, targeting bacteria in the respiratory tract. Eucalyptol's cooling effect soothes sore throats, eases breathing, and supports respiratory health naturally.

Add 2–3 drops of eucalyptus oil to hot water and inhale, or apply diluted oil to the chest.

Taking 600 mg of cineole (eucalyptol) daily may reduce COPD exacerbations by 38.5%.[51]

Try combining eucalyptus oil with peppermint for a stronger decongestant effect, enhanced sinus relief, and improved breathing.

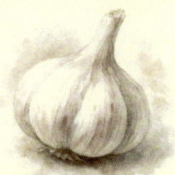

Garlic

Garlic's allicin boosts immune function and helps clear mucus naturally and effectively. Its antimicrobial properties target pathogens, reducing the duration and severity of colds and other respiratory issues. It's particularly effective at thinning mucus, easing congestion, and reducing cough frequency.

Consume 1-2 raw garlic cloves daily or add 1 teaspoon minced garlic to warm water or soups.

Daily garlic supplementation may reduce the frequency of colds by 63%.[52]

Crush garlic and let it sit for 10 minutes before use to boost its antimicrobial strength and immune-supporting benefits.

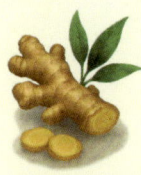

Ginger

Ginger's anti-inflammatory gingerols and shogaols soothe the respiratory tract, reducing inflammation and irritation. Its warming effect thins mucus, making it easier to expel, while its natural analgesic properties provide relief for sore throats, persistent coughing, and chest discomfort, promoting easier breathing.

Add 1 teaspoon of fresh grated ginger to hot water with honey, drink 2-3 times a day.

Taking 1.5 grams of ginger twice daily may shorten hospital stays for COVID-19 patients by 2.4 days.[53]

Pair ginger with lemon for added vitamin C to further boost immunity, enhance antioxidant protection, and support respiratory health.

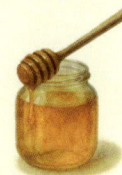

Honey

Honey coats and soothes the throat, reducing cough frequency and irritation. Its natural enzymes have antibacterial effects, helping to fight off respiratory infections. When combined with warm liquids, it becomes highly effective for relieving both dry and productive coughs and easing throat discomfort.

Take 1 tablespoon of raw honey, or mix with warm water and lemon, up to three times daily.

Honey may reduce cough frequency by 36% and severity by 44% in upper respiratory tract infections.[54]

Choose raw or unfiltered honey for the highest levels of antimicrobial enzymes, antioxidants, and natural healing properties.

Respiratory Health

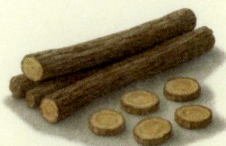

Licorice Root

Licorice root contains glycyrrhizin, which helps soothe inflamed airways, loosen mucus, and calm coughing. Its antiviral and anti-inflammatory properties also assist in respiratory infections. Known for its demulcent qualities, licorice coats the throat and eases irritation.

- Brew 1 teaspoon of dried licorice root in a cup of hot water, steep for 10 minutes, and drink 1-2 times a day.

- Glycyrrhizin from licorice root reduced asthma-related lung damage in mice, nearly matching a common asthma drug. [55]

- Avoid pairing with diuretics; licorice can significantly increase water retention when used with other compounds.

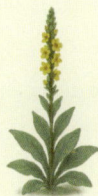

Mullein

Mullein is an expectorant herb, meaning it helps clear mucus from the lungs and airways. It also has anti-inflammatory properties that relieve irritation in the respiratory tract. Mullein's natural saponins promote lung detoxification by loosening and expelling mucus.

- Steep 1 tablespoon of dried mullein leaves in hot water for 10-15 minutes; drink 1-2 cups daily.

- In a trial of 200 acute bronchitis patients, a mullein extract reduced cough frequency by 53% after 7 days. [56]

- Strain mullein tea thoroughly to remove tiny leaf hairs, as they can cause throat irritation and discomfort when swallowed.

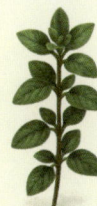

Oregano

Oregano contains carvacrol and thymol, potent compounds that fight respiratory bacterial and viral respiratory infections. It acts as a natural decongestant, clearing airways and easing sinus pressure. Oregano oil is especially effective at killing airborne pathogens and improving breathing.

- Use 1-2 drops of oregano oil in a diffuser for inhalation or add fresh oregano leaves to food.

- Patients with chronic rhinosinusitis using oregano oil nasal spray experienced a 51.52-point reduction in SNOT-22 scores. [57]

- Combine oregano oil with eucalyptus in a diffuser to enhance decongestant effects and improve breathing.

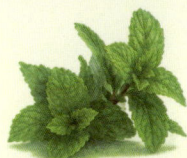

Peppermint

Peppermint contains menthol, which relaxes bronchial muscles and improves airflow. Its anti-inflammatory and antiviral properties support lung health, reduce inflammation, and help clear sinuses. It also acts as an expectorant, thinning mucus for easier removal and easing breathing discomfort effectively.

- Inhale peppermint oil or steep 1 tsp leaves in hot water for tea.

- Thirty students who took 0.05 ml peppermint oil in 500 mL water daily for 10 days showed better respiratory function. [58]

- Rub a drop of peppermint oil mixed with a carrier oil on the chest to naturally relieve chest congestion, open airways, and ease breathing.

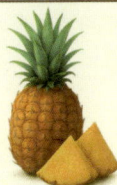

Pineapple

Pineapple contains bromelain, which has mucolytic properties—meaning it helps break down and thin mucus, making it easier to expel from the body. This can help reduce congestion, ease sinus pressure, support respiratory health, and improve overall breathing, comfort, and recovery from respiratory issues.

- Aim for approximately 360 ml (about 1.5 cups) of pineapple juice daily.

- Pineapple juice reduced mucus in plugs, suggesting it may help clear airways and reduce respiratory infection risk. [59]

- To maximize the benefits of pineapple juice, combine it with soothing ingredients like honey to support respiratory relief.

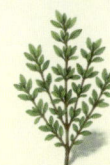

Thyme

Thyme is rich in thymol, a powerful antimicrobial that helps fight respiratory infections. It also acts as a natural decongestant and expectorant, clearing mucus and easing coughs. Its anti-inflammatory effects support lung health, improve airflow, and promote easier breathing.

- Steep 1 teaspoon of dried thyme in a cup of hot water for 10 minutes; drink 1-2 times a day.

- Thyme-primrose treatment reduced daytime coughing fits by 67.1% in acute bronchitis patients. [60]

- Add a few fresh thyme sprigs to steam inhalation for an enhanced decongestant effect, clearer sinuses, and improved respiratory relief.

Breathing & Lung Health

EXTRA HERBS

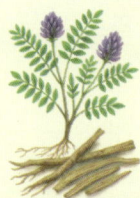

Astragalus

Astragalus is known for its immune-boosting effects and also supports respiratory health. It helps reduce inflammation in the lungs and enhances overall lung function.

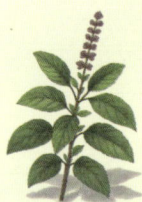

Holy Basil (Tulsi)

Holy Basil contains compounds that reduce lung inflammation and improve oxygen uptake. It supports respiratory function and helps enhance lung capacity naturally.

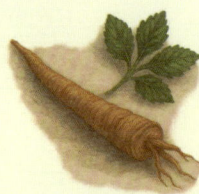

Marshmallow Root

Marshmallow root soothes the mucous membranes of the respiratory tract. It helps reduce irritation, support lung hydration, and promote easier breathing.

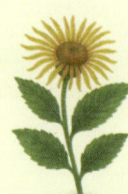

Elecampane

Elecampane acts as a natural expectorant that clears mucus from the lungs and improves airflow. It's valued for supporting respiratory function and relieving congestion.

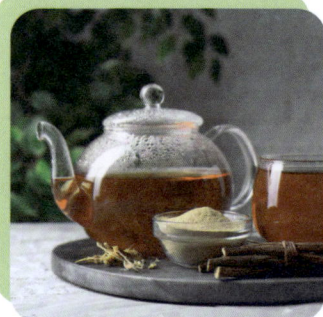

Lung-Boosting Ginger & Licorice Tea

This soothing tea combines ginger and licorice root to help support lung health. Ginger's anti-inflammatory properties work with licorice's soothing effects to help reduce inflammation and support easier breathing.

Ingredients:
- 1 tsp grated ginger
- 1 tsp dried licorice root
- 1 cup hot water
- 1 tsp honey (optional, for taste)

Instructions:
1. Add the ginger and licorice root to a cup of hot water.
2. Let it steep for 10 minutes.
3. Strain, add honey if desired, and enjoy warm.
4. Drink 1-2 times daily for best results.

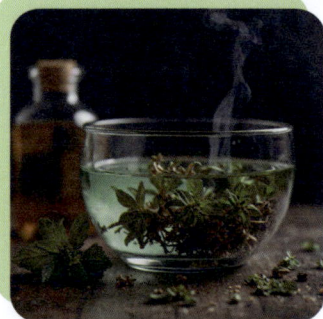

Peppermint & Thyme Steam Inhalation

This inhalation therapy combines peppermint and thyme to support clear breathing. Peppermint acts as a decongestant, while thyme's antimicrobial properties help eliminate respiratory pathogens.

Ingredients:
- 5 drops peppermint essential oil
- 1 tsp dried thyme
- 4 cups hot water

Instructions:
1. Boil water and pour it into a large bowl.
2. Add peppermint oil and thyme to the bowl.
3. Place a towel over your head and lean over the bowl, inhaling deeply for 5-10 minutes.
4. Use 1-2 times daily for relief and respiratory support.

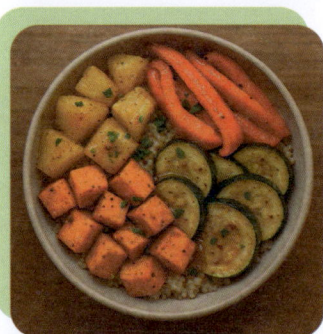

Roasted Pineapple, Honey & Ginger Veggie Bowls

This nourishing bowl features pineapple, rich in vitamin C and bromelain to support immune function and reduce inflammation. Ginger adds warmth and digestive support, while honey brings soothing antibacterial properties.

Ingredients (Serves 2):
- 1½ cups fresh pineapple chunks
- 1 medium sweet potato, cubed
- 1 red bell pepper, sliced
- 1 zucchini, sliced
- 1 tbsp olive oil
- Salt and pepper to taste
- ½ cup cooked quinoa, brown rice, or millet

For the glaze:
- 1 tbsp grated fresh ginger
- 2 tbsp raw honey
- 1 tbsp soy sauce or tamari
- Juice of ½ lime
- Optional: chili flakes for heat

Instructions:
1. Roast sweet potato, bell pepper, and zucchini at 200°C (400°F) for 25–30 mins.
2. Add pineapple for the last 10 mins.
3. Mix honey, ginger, soy sauce, and lime juice for the glaze.
4. Drizzle glaze over roasted mix and toss.
5. Serve warm over quinoa or rice.

Cough, Cold & Congestion

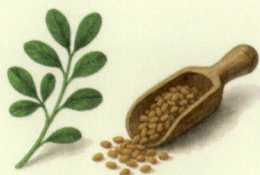

Fenugreek

Fenugreek contains saponins that help clear chest congestion and ease breathing. It has been shown to relieve symptoms of upper respiratory infections effectively.

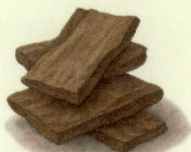

Slippery Elm

Slippery elm soothes the throat and respiratory tract by forming a protective mucilaginous layer. It reduces inflammation, eases irritation, and helps relieve cough and congestion naturally.

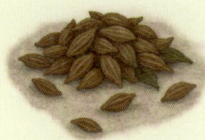

Anise Seed

Anise seed works as a natural expectorant and has antibacterial effects. It helps clear phlegm and provides relief from coughs and cold-related respiratory symptoms.

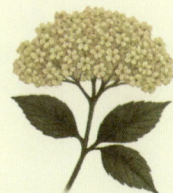

Elderflower

Elderflower is known for its antiviral and anti-inflammatory properties. It supports the immune system and helps reduce cold symptoms, including congestion and sinus pressure.

Cayenne & Honey Cough Syrup

Cayenne pepper boosts circulation and helps break up mucus, while honey soothes the throat and acts as a natural cough suppressant. Together, they make a powerful homemade cough syrup to relieve congestion and calm coughing spells.

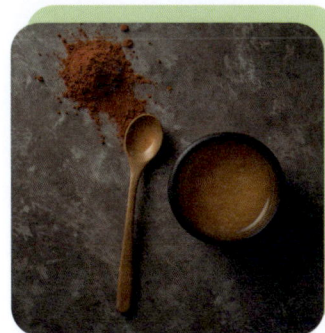

Ingredients:
- 1/4 tsp cayenne pepper
- 1 tbsp honey
- 1 tbsp apple cider vinegar
- Juice of 1 lemon
- 2 tbsp warm water

Instructions:
1. Mix all ingredients in a small bowl until well combined.
2. Take 1 teaspoon of the syrup every few hours as needed to soothe your throat and relieve coughing.
3. Store any leftover syrup in a small, sealed jar in the refrigerator for up to 2 days.

Mullein & Eucalyptus Chest Rub

This gentle, herbal chest rub uses mullein to soothe respiratory pathways, while eucalyptus oil opens airways and provides fast relief from congestion. Ideal for those nights when congestion interferes with restful sleep.

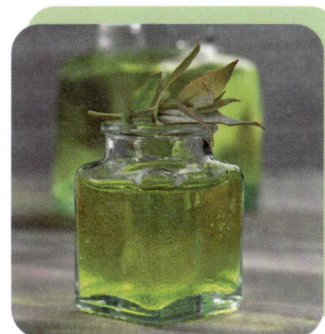

Ingredients:
- 1 tbsp dried mullein leaves (or 1 mullein tea bag)
- 1/4 cup coconut oil or olive oil
- 10 drops eucalyptus essential oil

Instructions:
1. Gently heat coconut or olive oil with mullein leaves for 10–15 mins.
2. Strain and pour infused oil into a jar.
3. Add eucalyptus oil and mix.
4. Apply to chest and throat as needed, especially before bed.

Garlic & Lemon Immunity Tonic

Garlic is a potent antimicrobial agent that helps fight infections, while lemon boosts the immune system with its high vitamin C content. This tonic is a quick way to bolster your defenses and reduce congestion.

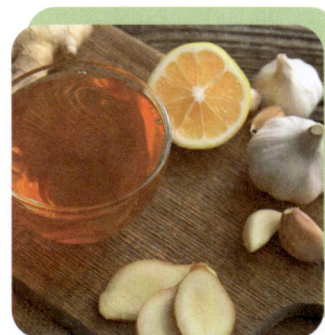

Ingredients:
- 1 clove garlic, minced
- Juice of 1 lemon
- 1 tsp honey
- 1 cup warm water

Instructions:
1. Add the minced garlic to the warm water and let steep for 5 minutes.
2. Strain the garlic if desired, then add the lemon juice and honey. Stir well.
3. Sip slowly and repeat up to twice daily during cold and flu season or whenever you're experiencing congestion.

Seasonal Allergies

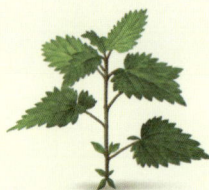

Stinging Nettle

Stinging nettle contains natural antihistamines and anti-inflammatory compounds. It helps reduce allergic reactions and relieves common symptoms like sneezing and itching.

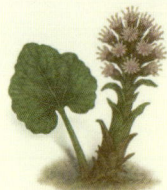

Butterbur

Butterbur has been shown to reduce allergy symptoms by inhibiting histamine release. It offers relief from nasal congestion, sneezing, and other seasonal allergy effects, promoting greater comfort.

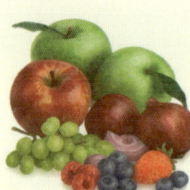

Quercetin

Quercetin is a natural flavonoid with strong antihistamine properties. It helps prevent histamine release, reducing symptoms like runny nose, itching, watery eyes, and sinus inflammation.

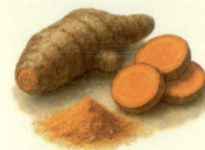

Turmeric

Turmeric contains curcumin, which has both anti-inflammatory and antihistamine effects. It helps reduce respiratory inflammation linked to allergies and eases breathing.

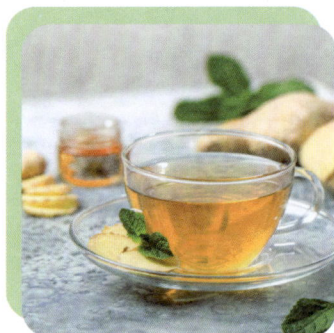

Peppermint & Ginger Anti-Allergy Tea

Peppermint contains rosmarinic acid, a compound known to reduce inflammation and relieve allergy symptoms, while ginger is a natural anti-inflammatory that can help ease nasal congestion and respiratory discomfort associated with allergies.

Ingredients:

- 1 tsp dried peppermint leaves (or 1 peppermint tea bag)
- 1-inch piece fresh ginger, sliced
- 1 cup hot water
- 1 tsp honey (optional, for taste)

Instructions:

1. Add the peppermint leaves and ginger slices to a cup of hot water and let steep for 5-10 minutes.
2. Strain, add honey if desired, and sip slowly.
3. Drink up to twice daily to help manage allergy symptoms.

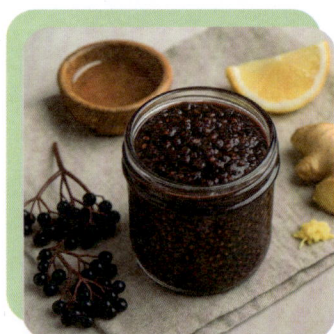

Immune-Boosting Elderberry Chia Jam

Elderberries are packed with antioxidants that may reduce cold and flu severity. Paired with fiber-rich chia seeds and soothing raw honey, this recipe supports immunity, gut health, and inflammation relief.

Ingredients (Makes ~1 cup):

- 1 cup fresh/frozen elderberries (or ½ cup dried, rehydrated)
- 2 tbsp chia seeds
- 2–3 tbsp water
- 1–2 tsp raw honey (to taste)
- ½ tsp grated ginger (optional)
- Squeeze of lemon juice (optional)

Instructions:

1. Simmer elderberries and water for 8–10 mins until soft.
2. Mash slightly, add chia seeds and optional ginger.
3. Simmer 2–3 more mins to thicken.
4. Cool slightly, then stir in honey and lemon juice.
5. Chill in a jar for 1–2 hours to set.

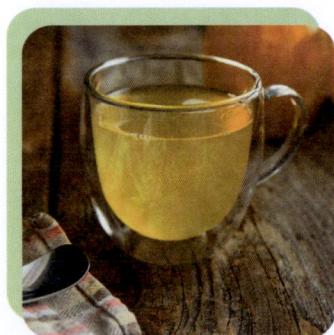

Apple Cider Vinegar & Honey Allergy Tonic

Apple cider vinegar helps balance the body's pH levels and reduce mucus production, making it a helpful remedy for seasonal allergies. Combined with honey, it soothes the throat and supports immune health.

Ingredients:

- 1 tbsp apple cider vinegar
- 1 tbsp honey (preferably raw and local)
- 1 cup warm water

Instructions:

1. Mix apple cider vinegar and honey in warm water until fully dissolved.
2. Drink once daily in the morning for optimal results during allergy season.

Sinus Health

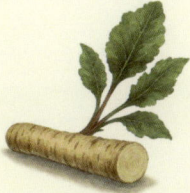

Horseradish

Horseradish acts as a natural decongestant by breaking down mucus. It helps clear nasal passages, reduce sinus pressure, relieve congestion, and improve overall airflow and breathing comfort.

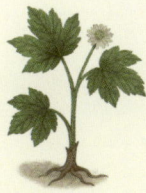

Goldenseal

Goldenseal is known for its antimicrobial and anti-inflammatory effects. It helps fight sinus infections, reduces swelling in the nasal and sinus passages, and supports faster recovery and clearer breathing.

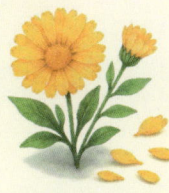

Calendula

Calendula contains compounds that reduce inflammation and fight microbes. It soothes irritated sinuses and helps prevent infection and congestion-related discomfort.

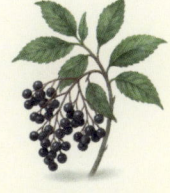

Elderberry

Elderberry has antiviral and anti-inflammatory properties that support respiratory health. It helps reduce sinus swelling, clear mucus, relieve congestion and pressure, and strengthen natural defenses against infections.

Eucalyptus & Peppermint Steam Inhalation

Eucalyptus and peppermint oils are known for their powerful decongestant properties, helping to open the sinus passages and relieve sinus pressure. Inhalation therapy with these oils can provide quick, effective relief from sinus congestion.

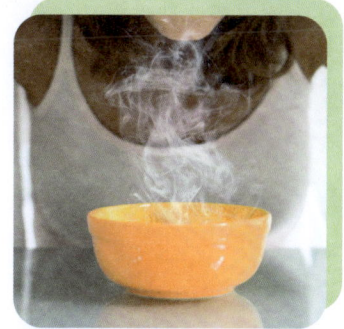

Ingredients:

- 4 cups boiling water
- 5 drops eucalyptus essential oil
- 3 drops peppermint essential oil

Instructions:

1. Pour boiling water into a large, heat-safe bowl.
2. Add eucalyptus and peppermint oils to the water.
3. Lean over the bowl, draping a towel over your head to trap the steam.
4. Inhale deeply for 5-10 minutes, taking breaks as needed. Repeat once or twice daily for relief.

Garlic & Cayenne Sinus-Clearing Tonic

Garlic's natural antibacterial properties and cayenne's ability to stimulate circulation make this tonic a powerful remedy for clearing out sinus blockages and fighting infection.

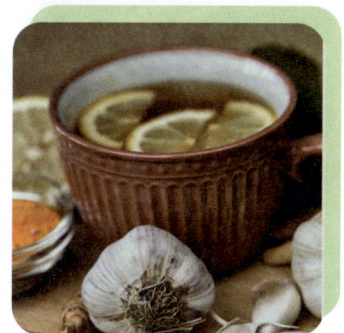

Ingredients:

- 1 clove garlic, minced
- 1/4 tsp cayenne pepper
- Juice of 1 lemon
- 1 cup warm water

Instructions:

1. Add minced garlic and cayenne pepper to a cup of warm water.
2. Squeeze in the lemon juice and stir well.
3. Drink slowly, allowing the tonic to work on clearing sinus passages. Use once daily during sinus flare-ups.

Thyme & Garlic Sinus-Clearing Soup

Thyme, a natural expectorant, clears mucus, while garlic's antimicrobial properties combat infections. This flavorful soup is a comforting remedy for sinus congestion.

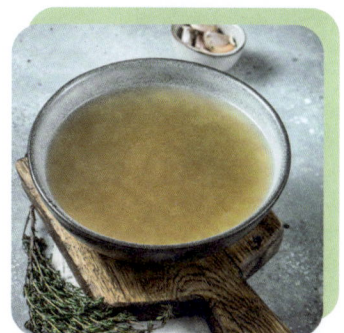

Ingredients:

- 2 cups vegetable or chicken broth
- 1 tsp dried thyme (or a handful of fresh thyme sprigs)
- 2 cloves garlic, minced
- Juice of 1/2 lemon
- Salt and pepper to taste

Instructions:

1. Bring the broth to a simmer in a pot over medium heat.
2. Add thyme and minced garlic, simmer for 10 minutes.
3. Remove from heat, add lemon juice, and season with salt and pepper.
4. Enjoy the soup warm, sipping slowly to allow the steam to help clear your sinuses. Use as a meal or remedy once daily.

Blood Sugar

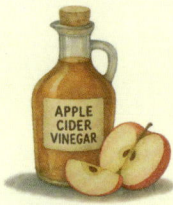

Apple Cider Vinegar

The acetic acid in apple cider vinegar slows the breakdown of starches into sugars, significantly lowering blood sugar spikes after meals. It also improves insulin sensitivity, especially after carbohydrate-rich meals, which is key for effectively managing diabetes.

🍽 Mix 1 tablespoon in water before meals or add to salad dressings.

⚗ Daily intake of apple cider vinegar may lower fasting blood sugar by approximately 8 mg/dL.[61]

🌿 Choose raw, unfiltered apple cider vinegar for best results, and always dilute it to protect tooth enamel and support safe daily use.

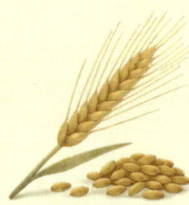

Barley

Barley is rich in β-glucan, a type of soluble fiber that slows digestion and helps prevent sharp spikes in blood sugar after meals. It also improves the body's insulin response, making it easier for the body to consistently manage glucose levels over time.

🍽 Aim for ½ to 1 cup of cooked barley daily to get 3–6 g of β-glucan, supporting healthy blood sugar.

⚗ One study found that barley lowered post-meal blood sugar by up to 65% and insulin by 56%, outperforming oats and glucose.[62]

🌿 Swap white rice with hulled or pearl barley in meals to help stabilize your blood sugar naturally and support long-term metabolic health.

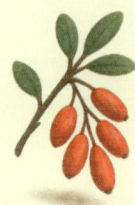

Berberine

Found in plants like goldenseal and barberry, berberine activates enzymes that help cells take up glucose and reduce glucose production in the liver. It also improves lipid profiles and insulin sensitivity, contributing to overall metabolic health and balance.

🍽 Take 500 mg of berberine twice daily with meals.

⚗ Berberine supplements may lower fasting blood sugar by about 15 mg/dL in people with type 2 diabetes.[63]

🌿 Berberine works synergistically with milk thistle, boosting liver protection, enhancing antioxidant activity, and aiding digestion.

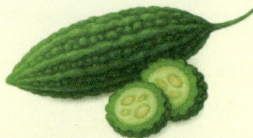

Bitter Melon

Bitter melon contains compounds that mimic insulin, helping cells take up glucose more efficiently. It also enhances insulin production and improves glycogen storage, steadily reducing overall blood sugar levels in the bloodstream over time, supporting metabolic balance and energy regulation.

🍽 Drink 1/2 cup of bitter melon juice or take 500 mg of extract daily.

⚗ Taking 2 g of bitter melon daily may reduce fasting blood sugar by about 15 mg/dL in type 2 diabetes.[64]

🌿 Soak the melon in salt water for several minutes to reduce bitterness before juicing or cooking, making it more palatable and easier to enjoy.

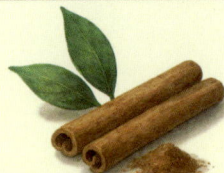

Cinnamon

Cinnamon contains compounds that enhance insulin receptor function and help increase glucose transport into cells. Its active compound, cinnamaldehyde, also has anti-inflammatory effects that support overall metabolic health, stabilize blood sugar, and promote better energy utilization.

🍽 Add 1/2 to 1 teaspoon daily to oatmeal, smoothies, or tea.

⚗ Taking cinnamon supplements may lower fasting blood sugar by about 25 mg/dL in people with type 2 diabetes.[65]

🌿 Use Ceylon cinnamon ("true" cinnamon) as it is safer for long-term use and has a milder flavor than cassia cinnamon.

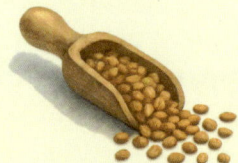

Fenugreek Seeds

Rich in soluble fiber, fenugreek seeds slow carbohydrate absorption, preventing blood sugar spikes after meals. They also enhance insulin release and sensitivity, which aids in long-term diabetes management and improves cholesterol levels for better heart health and stability.

🍽 Soak 1-2 tablespoons in water overnight and drink on an empty stomach in the morning.

⚗ Incorporating fenugreek seeds into your diet may lower fasting blood sugar by about 17 mg/dL.[66]

🌿 Crush the seeds before soaking to boost their benefits. Fenugreek also pairs well with ginger to support better digestion and reduce bloating.

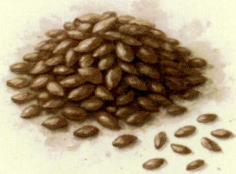

Blood Sugar

Flaxseeds

Flaxseeds are rich in fiber and lignans, compounds that help slow the absorption of sugars, effectively preventing spikes in blood sugar levels. The alpha-linolenic acid in flax also reduces inflammation, which supports overall insulin sensitivity and metabolic balance.

- Consume 1 tablespoon of ground flaxseed daily, mixed into smoothies, oatmeal, or yogurt.

- Adding 10 g of flaxseed powder daily may cut fasting blood sugar by nearly 20% in type 2 diabetes.[67]

- Grind flaxseeds fresh to preserve nutrients, and store in the refrigerator to prevent them from going rancid.

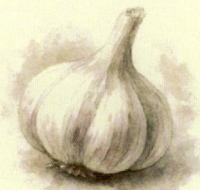

Garlic

Garlic contains sulfur compounds that improve insulin sensitivity, making cells more responsive to insulin. It also supports heart health, which is particularly beneficial for diabetics. Regular garlic intake has shown a modest but consistent blood sugar-lowering effect.

- Eat 1-2 raw cloves daily or add minced garlic to meals.

- Adding garlic supplements to your diet may lower fasting blood sugar by about 7 mg/dL in type 2 diabetes.[68]

- Crush garlic and let it sit for 10 minutes before eating to boost its active compounds.

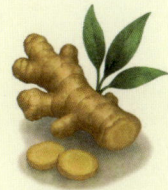

Ginger

Ginger helps regulate insulin and enhances glucose uptake in cells, effectively lowering blood sugar levels. It also reduces inflammation, which can improve insulin sensitivity and support more stable blood sugar control over time for better metabolic health.

- Take 1-2 grams of fresh ginger daily in teas, smoothies, or added to meals.

- Taking 2 grams of ginger daily may lower fasting blood sugar by 12% in people with type 2 diabetes.[69]

- Combine ginger with a pinch of cinnamon to boost anti-diabetic effects. Both work synergistically for blood sugar control.

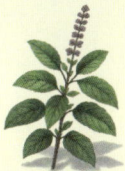

Holy Basil

Holy Basil, also known as Tulsi, has powerful adaptogenic properties that help lower cortisol levels, which in turn helps stabilize blood sugar levels naturally. Its active compounds support improved insulin function and may help reduce fasting blood glucose levels over time, promoting overall metabolic balance and resilience.

- Consume 1-2 cups of holy basil tea daily or take fresh leaves as a garnish.

- Incorporating holy basil into your routine may lower fasting blood sugar by about 17% in people with type 2 diabetes.[70]

- Use fresh holy basil leaves when possible, as they contain more active compounds than dried ones, offering greater therapeutic health benefits.

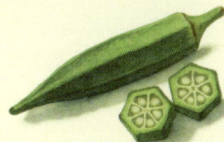

Okra

Okra contains soluble fiber that slows sugar absorption and flavonoids that help reduce blood sugar levels. Its mucilage, a gel-like substance, has shown promising effects in improving glycemic control over time, supporting insulin sensitivity and promoting long-term metabolic health naturally and effectively.

- Consume 100 grams of cooked okra daily. Soak cut okra in water overnight and drink it in the morning.

- Incorporating okra into your diet may lower fasting blood sugar by about 10 mg/dL in people with type 2 diabetes.[71]

- For a stronger effect, soak sliced okra overnight and drink the water to extract its beneficial compounds.

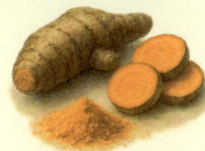

Turmeric

Turmeric contains curcumin, which enhances insulin sensitivity and exerts anti-inflammatory effects that support healthy glucose metabolism. It also aids in reducing oxidative stress, a key factor in the development and progression of diabetes and other metabolic-related chronic health conditions.

- Add 1/2 teaspoon of turmeric powder to meals daily, ideally combined with black pepper to improve absorption.

- Incorporating turmeric into your diet may lower fasting blood sugar by about 8 mg/dL in people with type 2 diabetes.[72]

- Pair turmeric with a healthy fat, like olive oil or coconut oil, for optimal absorption and enhanced blood sugar benefits.

Diabetes Management

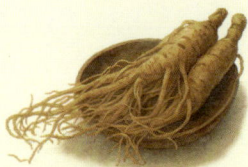

Ginseng

Ginseng contains ginsenosides, which help stabilize blood sugar by enhancing insulin sensitivity and reducing post-meal glucose spikes, supporting overall glycemic control.

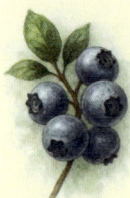

Blueberry

Blueberries are rich in anthocyanins, which improve glucose metabolism and reduce inflammation. They support blood sugar balance and aid in managing diabetes naturally.

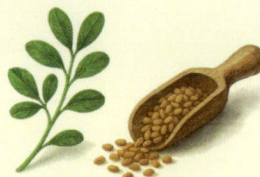

Fenugreek Leaves

Fenugreek leaves contain compounds that slow carbohydrate absorption and improve glucose tolerance, effective in managing blood sugar levels without medication.

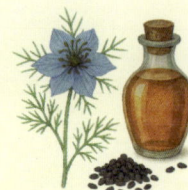

Nigella Sativa (Black Seed)

Nigella sativa contains thymoquinone, which may reduce fasting blood sugar and enhance pancreatic beta-cell function, supporting insulin production and glucose control.

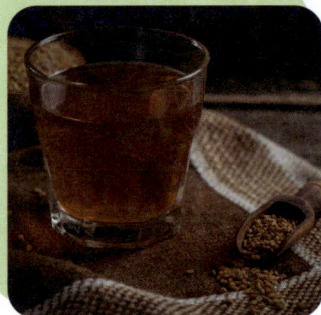

Cinnamon Fenugreek Tea

Cinnamon and fenugreek seeds have been shown to help regulate blood sugar levels by enhancing insulin sensitivity and reducing fasting blood glucose. This tea combines these powerful ingredients to create an effective and tasty way to support blood sugar control.

Ingredients:

- 1 cup hot water
- 1/2 tsp cinnamon powder
- 1 tsp fenugreek seeds, lightly crushed
- 1 tsp lemon juice (optional)

Instructions:

1. Add the fenugreek seeds to hot water and let steep for 5-10 minutes.
2. Stir in the cinnamon powder and let sit for an additional 2 minutes.
3. Strain and add lemon juice if desired.
4. Drink warm, preferably on an empty stomach in the morning, for best results.

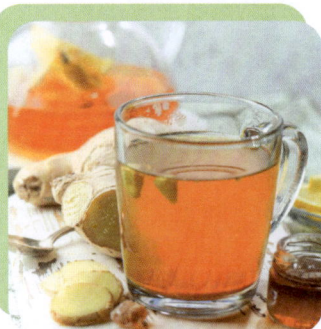

Apple Cider Vinegar & Ginger Elixir

Apple cider vinegar and ginger have shown to help improve insulin sensitivity and lower blood sugar spikes after meals. This refreshing elixir is easy to incorporate daily for stable blood sugar levels.

Ingredients:

- 1 tbsp apple cider vinegar
- 1 cup water
- 1 tsp grated ginger
- A pinch of cinnamon (optional for taste)

Instructions:

1. Mix apple cider vinegar and water in a glass.
2. Add grated ginger and stir well. Add a pinch of cinnamon if you prefer.
3. Let it sit for 2-3 minutes for flavors to blend.
4. Drink before meals to aid in blood sugar control.

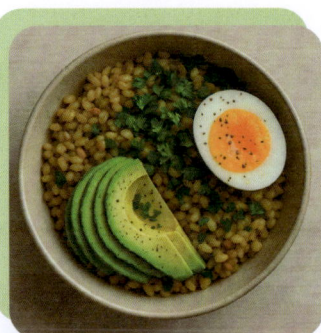

Barley & Fenugreek Savory Breakfast Bowl

Barley's beta-glucan fiber and fenugreek's blood sugar–lowering effects help slow digestion and improve insulin response. Paired with protein and healthy fats, this makes a balanced, low-glycemic meal for steady energy.

Ingredients:

- ¾ cup pearl or hulled barley
- 1 tbsp fenugreek seeds
- 2 soft-boiled/poached eggs (optional)
- ½ avocado, sliced
- 1 tbsp olive oil or ghee
- ½ tsp turmeric
- Salt & pepper to taste
- Chopped parsley or cilantro (garnish)
- Optional: sautéed greens, roasted veggies, or Greek yogurt

Instructions:

1. Cook barley with fenugreek seeds until tender (25–40 mins).
2. Drain and season with turmeric, oil, salt, and pepper.
3. Serve warm topped with egg, avocado, and herbs.
4. Add optional greens or yogurt for extra nutrients.

Insulin & Blood Sugar Balancing

EXTRA HERBS

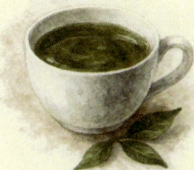

Green Tea

Green tea is rich in polyphenols, especially catechins, which help improve insulin sensitivity and support long-term reductions in blood glucose levels beneficial to a diabetes-friendly lifestyle.

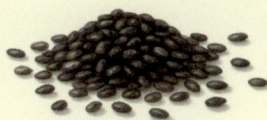

Chia Seeds

Chia seeds are high in fiber and omega-3 fatty acids, which help slow digestion, stabilize blood sugar levels, and support a balanced insulin response throughout the day for improved metabolic health.

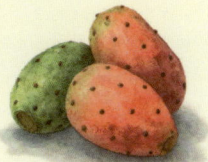

Prickly Pear

Prickly pear is known for its blood sugar-lowering effects. Its rich fiber and pectin content help slow carbohydrate absorption, reduce post-meal glucose spikes, and improve insulin sensitivity for better metabolic control.

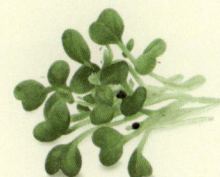

Broccoli Sprouts

Broccoli sprouts contain sulforaphane, a compound shown to lower blood sugar and improve insulin resistance, making them especially beneficial for diabetes management.

Cinnamon & Flaxseed Smoothie

Cinnamon helps enhance insulin sensitivity, while flaxseeds provide fiber and omega-3s, making this smoothie a blood sugar-friendly option to keep you full and energized without spikes.

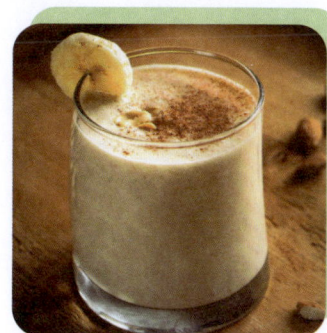

Ingredients:
- 1 cup unsweetened coconut milk (or other plant-based milk)
- 1 tsp cinnamon powder
- 1 tbsp ground flaxseeds
- 1/2 banana (for natural sweetness)
- A few ice cubes (optional)

Instructions:
1. Combine all ingredients in a blender and blend until smooth.
2. Pour into a glass and enjoy as a morning or midday snack.
3. Drink immediately to preserve the nutrients and flavors.

Bitter Melon & Apple Cider Vinegar Tonic

Bitter melon is known for its active compounds that mimic insulin, while apple cider vinegar helps stabilize blood sugar, making this tonic a strong ally for maintaining balanced blood sugar.

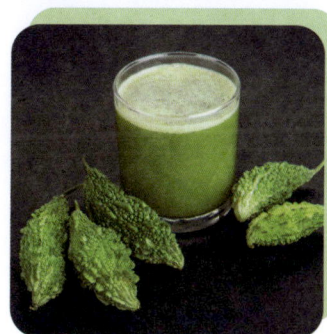

Ingredients:
- 1 small bitter melon, deseeded and chopped
- 1 tbsp apple cider vinegar
- 1 cup water
- 1 tsp honey (optional for taste)

Instructions:
1. Blend the bitter melon with water until smooth, then strain to remove pulp.
2. Add apple cider vinegar and honey if desired, stirring well.
3. Drink in the morning on an empty stomach or before meals to help improve insulin sensitivity.

Blueberry, Cinnamon & Chia Pudding

Chia seeds, blueberries, and cinnamon work together to support blood sugar balance. Chia offers fiber and omega-3s, blueberries boost insulin sensitivity, and cinnamon enhances glucose control for steady energy and fullness.

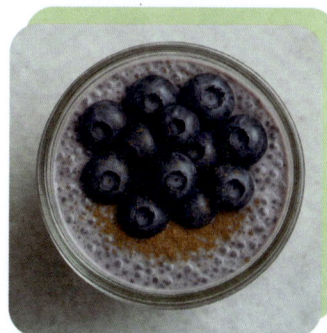

Ingredients (Serves 1–2):
- 3 tbsp chia seeds
- ¾ cup unsweetened almond milk (or milk of choice)
- ½ cup fresh or frozen blueberries
- ½ tsp ground cinnamon
- 1 tsp vanilla extract (optional)
- 1–2 tsp ground flaxseed (optional, for extra fiber)
- 1 tsp honey or stevia (optional, adjust to taste)

Instructions:
1. Mix chia seeds, almond milk, cinnamon, and vanilla in a jar. Stir well.
2. Add blueberries and stir gently.
3. Cover and chill for at least 2 hours or overnight.
4. Stir before serving. Top with berries, cinnamon, or walnuts if desired.

Metabolic Health

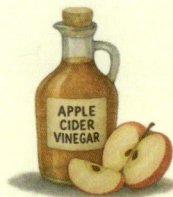

Apple Cider Vinegar

Apple cider vinegar (ACV) contains acetic acid, which helps improve metabolism by increasing enzyme activity, aiding in fat breakdown, and balancing blood sugar levels. ACV also promotes a feeling of fullness, reducing calorie intake and curbing sugar cravings.

- Mix 1-2 teaspoons of ACV in a glass of water before meals, up to 2 times daily.

- Daily intake of 1 tablespoon of ACV for 3 months led to an average 15-pound weight loss in overweight youth.[73]

- Look for raw, unfiltered ACV with "the mother" for optimal health benefits, as it contains beneficial enzymes and probiotics.

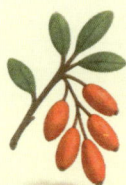

Berberine

Helps regulate blood sugar, improves insulin sensitivity, and activates AMPK—an enzyme that boosts fat burning and energy use. It also reduces glucose production in the liver and may help lower HbA1c levels, supporting long-term metabolic health and diabetes management.

- 500 mg, 2–3 times per day with meals (totaling 1000–1500 mg daily) is the typical effective dose.

- Berberine improved body shape and metabolism in women with PCOS, reducing waist size more than metformin or placebo.[74]

- Take berberine with meals to enhance its blood sugar–lowering effects and reduce the chance of stomach upset.

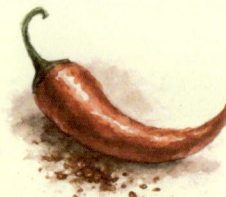

Cayenne Pepper

Cayenne pepper contains capsaicin, a natural compound that boosts metabolism by inducing thermogenesis, increasing calorie expenditure, and reducing appetite. It also helps in breaking down fat cells, supporting healthy weight management and metabolic health overall.

- Add 1/8 teaspoon of cayenne pepper to meals or mix in a warm beverage once daily.

- Daily intake of 4 milligrams of capsaicin for three months reduced body fat percentage.[75]

- Start with a small amount if you're sensitive to spice, and gradually increase the quantity to build tolerance and avoid digestive discomfort.

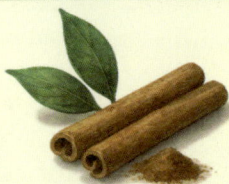

Cinnamon

Cinnamon is rich in polyphenols that help regulate blood sugar, reducing insulin spikes and keeping energy levels steady. It also curbs cravings for sweets and promotes fat metabolism, aiding in weight management and supporting long-term metabolic and hormonal health with consistent use.

- Use 1/2 to 1 teaspoon of Ceylon cinnamon powder daily, in smoothies, teas, or meals.

- Cinnamon supplements significantly lower weight and BMI, especially at doses of 3 g or more daily.[76]

- Opt for Ceylon cinnamon, known as "true cinnamon," for higher antioxidant content and a sweeter flavor.

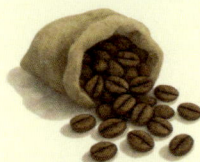

Coffee

Coffee contains caffeine, a natural stimulant that activates the central nervous system, boosting metabolic rate and enhancing fat oxidation. It also provides a quick energy lift, helping to reduce fatigue, sharpen mental focus, and support improved physical performance and endurance throughout the day.

- Consume 1-2 cups of black coffee daily, ideally without added sugar or cream.

- One extra cup of unsweetened coffee daily may lead to about 0.26 pounds of weight loss over four years.[77]

- Drink coffee before exercise to enhance fat burn and endurance, as caffeine helps release fatty acids for energy use.

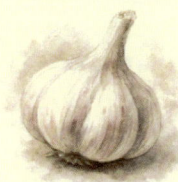

Garlic

Garlic contains bioactive compounds that stimulate the breakdown of fats and promote thermogenesis, helping to boost metabolic rate naturally and efficiently. Its sulfur compounds also assist in managing insulin levels, which can reduce fat accumulation and support long-term weight control.

- Consume 1-2 raw cloves daily or add 1 teaspoon of chopped garlic to meals.

- Garlic extract helped reduce weight and improve insulin resistance in obese women, with small changes in gut bacteria.[78]

- Try aged garlic, as it retains antioxidant properties without the intense odor of fresh garlic.

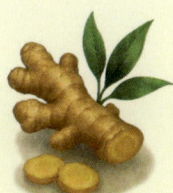

Metabolic Health

Ginger

Ginger has compounds like gingerol that enhance thermogenesis, raising body temperature and helping to burn more calories. It also regulates blood sugar and curbs appetite, reducing cravings. Additionally, it aids digestion, reducing bloating and discomfort.

Add 1-2 teaspoons of grated ginger to hot water or tea daily.

Adding ginger to your diet may lead to about 1.5 pounds of weight loss and a lower waist-to-hip ratio.[79]

Combine ginger with green tea for an added metabolism-boosting effect and improved fat oxidation.

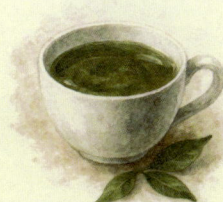

Green Tea

Green tea contains catechins and caffeine, which work together to increase fat oxidation and energy expenditure. These compounds help the body burn more calories during and after exercise, assisting in weight loss, improving metabolic efficiency, and supporting long-term energy balance.

Drink 2-3 cups of green tea per day, ideally before exercise.

Regular green tea intake may result in a minimal weight loss of approximately 0.09 pounds over three months.[80]

Add a squeeze of lemon to green tea to enhance catechin absorption and boost its metabolism-enhancing effects.

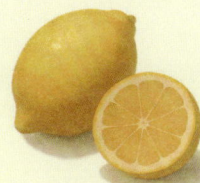

Lemon

Lemon is rich in vitamin C and polyphenols, which aid in detoxifying the liver and enhancing fat metabolism. Its sour taste can help reduce sugar cravings, and drinking lemon juice in water supports hydration—an essential factor for optimal metabolic function and overall energy balance.

Add juice of half a lemon to warm water and drink in the morning.

Consuming warm lemon water before breakfast and dinner may result in a weight loss of 2 to 9 pounds over three weeks.[81]

Pair lemon with green tea to increase the absorption of antioxidants and support fat loss.

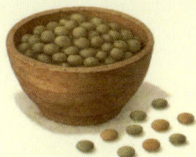

Lentils

Legumes are high in protein, fiber, and resistant starch, which help you feel full longer, reduce appetite, and support steady blood sugar levels throughout the day. Also, they may boost mitochondrial activity, helping the body burn energy more efficiently and sustain metabolic health over time.

Aim for 1 to 1½ cups of cooked legumes per day to support weight and metabolic health.

A low-calorie, legume-rich diet caused 8.3% weight loss in 8 weeks, matching high-protein and beating standard diets.[82]

Swap out refined carbs like pasta for legumes, they keep you full longer and support fat-burning without added calories.

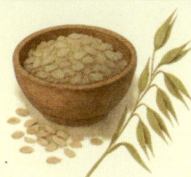

Oats

Oats are high in beta-glucan, a type of soluble fiber that slows digestion, stabilizes blood sugar levels, and helps keep you feeling full for longer. This can aid in weight management and reduce overall calorie intake. Additionally, it supports metabolic health, improves cholesterol levels, and promotes overall digestive wellness.

Consume 1/2 cup of oats as part of breakfast or as a snack.

Oats significantly lowered fasting insulin by 6.29 pmol/L and reduced glucose AUC by 30.23 min×mmol/L.[83]

Add cinnamon to your oats for a natural metabolism boost and enhanced blood sugar control.

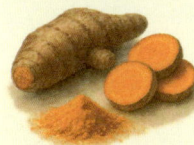

Turmeric

Turmeric's active compound, curcumin, has been shown to reduce inflammation and support fat breakdown, making it beneficial for weight loss and overall metabolism. Curcumin also promotes healthy liver function, which is crucial for detoxifying the body, balancing hormones, and effectively managing body weight.

Take 1/2 teaspoon of turmeric with a pinch of black pepper daily, in water or as part of meals.

Curcumin reduced BMI by 0.37, weight by 0.23 kg, waist by 0.25 cm, and raised adiponectin by 1.05 µg/mL.[84]

Pair turmeric with black pepper to enhance curcumin absorption by up to 2000%, maximizing its metabolic benefits.

Boosting Metabolism

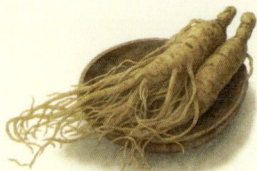

Ginseng

Ginseng contains ginsenosides that enhance energy metabolism by promoting fat oxidation and thermogenesis, making it a powerful natural metabolic booster.

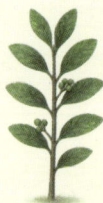

Yerba Mate

Yerba mate is rich in caffeine and antioxidants that stimulate metabolism and support fat oxidation, helping the body burn calories more efficiently throughout the day and enhancing overall energy levels.

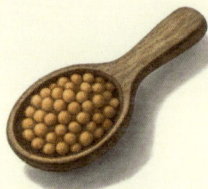

Mustard Seeds

Mustard seeds contain glucosinolates, which may increase metabolic rate and promote calorie burn. They're a beneficial addition to natural metabolism-enhancing strategies.

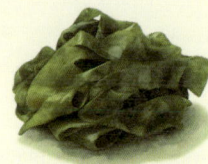

Seaweed (Kelp)

Seaweed is high in iodine, a mineral essential for proper thyroid function. A healthy thyroid supports optimal metabolic rate and energy production, which play a key role in maintaining weight balance.

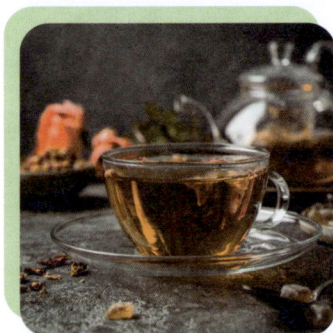

Spicy Metabolism-Boosting Tea

Green tea is rich in catechins and caffeine, which are known to enhance thermogenesis, aiding the body in burning calories. Cayenne pepper contains capsaicin, which increases metabolic rate, while lemon provides antioxidants and vitamin C to support cellular energy production.

Ingredients:
- 1 cup hot water
- 1 green tea bag
- 1/4 tsp cayenne pepper
- Juice of 1/2 lemon

Instructions:
1. Steep the green tea bag in hot water for 3-5 minutes, then remove the bag.
2. Stir in the cayenne pepper and lemon juice until well mixed.
3. Sip slowly, ideally in the morning or before a workout, to enjoy a metabolism boost.

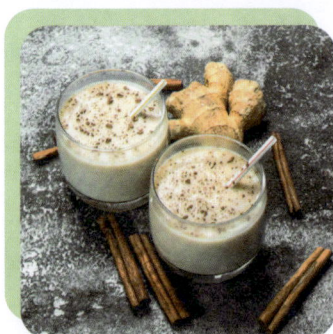

Ginger-Cinnamon Morning Smoothie

Ginger and cinnamon both stimulate the metabolism and help regulate blood sugar levels, which can prevent energy crashes and support fat metabolism. Oats add fiber to keep you full, helping curb cravings throughout the day.

Ingredients:
- 1/2 cup rolled oats
- 1/2 tsp ground cinnamon
- 1/2 tsp grated ginger (or 1/4 tsp ground ginger)
- 1 cup almond milk (or any milk of choice)
- 1/2 banana (optional, for added sweetness)

Instructions:
1. Blend all ingredients together until smooth.
2. Pour into a glass and enjoy as a breakfast smoothie or a metabolism-boosting snack.

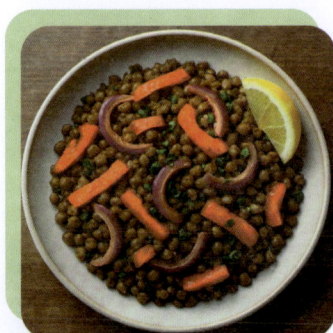

Spicy Garlic Lentil Stir-Fry

Lentils provide fiber and protein to curb cravings and regulate blood sugar. Garlic aids metabolism, and cayenne boosts calorie burn and reduces hunger—making this a satisfying, weight-friendly meal.

Ingredients:
- 1 cup cooked green/brown lentils
- 1 tbsp olive or avocado oil
- 3 garlic cloves, minced
- 1/2 red onion, sliced
- 1 bell pepper, chopped
- 1 tsp cumin
- 1/4–1/2 tsp cayenne (to taste)
- Salt & pepper to taste
- Juice of 1/2 lemon
- Fresh parsley or cilantro (garnish)

Instructions:
1. Sauté garlic and red onion in oil for 2–3 mins.
2. Add bell pepper; cook 3–4 mins until soft.
3. Stir in lentils, cumin, cayenne, salt, and pepper.
4. Cook 5–7 mins, stirring, until heated through and lightly crisped.

Weight Loss & Appetite Control

EXTRA HERBS

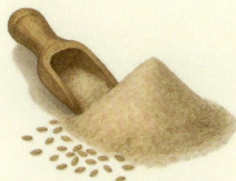

Psyllium Husk

Psyllium husk is a high-fiber ingredient that promotes fullness and appetite regulation. It supports portion control and can help reduce overall calorie intake for weight loss.

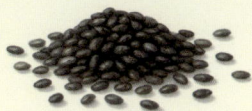

Chia Seeds

Chia seeds are rich in fiber and omega-3 fatty acids. They absorb liquid and expand in the stomach, creating a lasting feeling of fullness that helps curb appetite, reduce overeating, and support weight management.

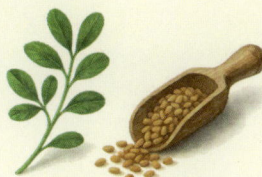

Fenugreek

Fenugreek seeds contain fiber that supports appetite control and helps stabilize blood sugar. This dual action can contribute to reduced calorie intake and healthy weight loss.

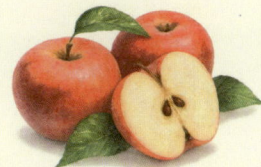

Apple

Apples are high in fiber and water, promoting a lasting sense of fullness. Their natural polyphenols may also aid in fat metabolism and support long-term weight management and overall health.

Lemon-Ginger Appetite Control Drink

Lemon and ginger work synergistically to aid digestion, regulate blood sugar, and curb appetite. Ginger is known to reduce hunger and promote satiety, while lemon's pectin fiber helps you feel fuller longer, reducing unnecessary snacking.

Ingredients:
- 1 cup warm water
- 1/2 lemon, juiced
- 1/2 tsp grated fresh ginger (or 1/4 tsp ground ginger)
- A dash of cayenne pepper (optional for metabolism boost)

Instructions:
1. Combine all ingredients in a cup and stir well.
2. Drink this first thing in the morning or between meals to help control appetite.

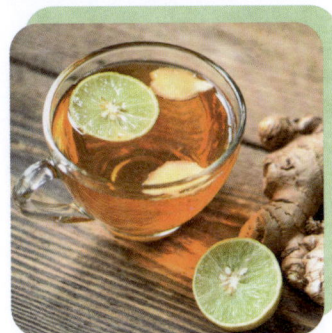

Cinnamon-Oat Smoothie Bowl

Cinnamon helps stabilize blood sugar levels, reducing cravings, while oats provide fiber and protein, promoting fullness. This smoothie bowl is a satisfying, nutrient-dense option for breakfast or a snack that can help curb hunger throughout the day.

Ingredients:
- 1/2 cup rolled oats
- 1/2 cup almond milk (or milk of choice)
- 1/2 banana (for natural sweetness)
- 1/2 tsp ground cinnamon
- A handful of berries (optional for added flavor and nutrients)

Instructions:
1. Blend oats, milk, banana, and cinnamon until smooth.
2. Pour into a bowl, top with berries, and enjoy as a filling meal to help control appetite.

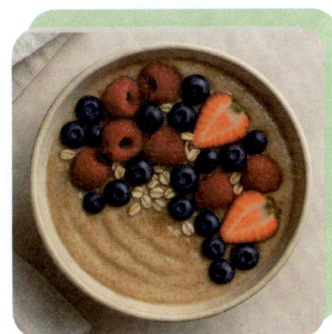

Apple Pie Overnight Oats

This filling breakfast supports weight management with fiber-rich oats and apples, blood sugar–balancing cinnamon, and metabolism-boosting ginger—for steady energy and reduced cravings.

Ingredients:
- ½ cup rolled oats
- ½ apple, diced (with skin)
- ¾ cup almond milk (or any milk)
- ½ tsp cinnamon
- ¼ tsp ginger
- 1 tsp chia seeds (optional)
- ½ tsp vanilla (optional)
- 1–2 tsp honey or stevia (optional)
- Pinch of salt
- Optional toppings: a few chopped walnuts or a spoon of plain Greek yogurt

Instructions:
1. Mix oats, apple, cinnamon, ginger, chia seeds, and salt in a jar.
2. Add milk, vanilla (if using), and sweetener. Stir well.
3. Cover and refrigerate overnight (or 6+ hours).
4. Stir in the morning and top with walnuts or yogurt. Enjoy cold or warmed.

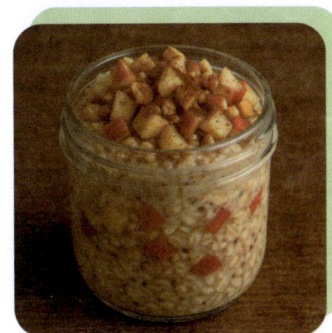

Energy & Fatigue Management

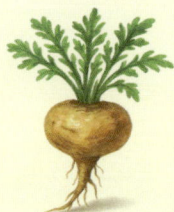

Maca Root

Maca root is an adaptogen known for naturally enhancing energy without causing jitters or crashes. It supports stamina, balances hormones, and helps maintain steady energy levels throughout the day.

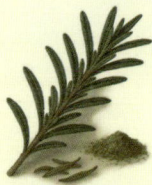

Rosemary

Rosemary enhances our energy by improving blood circulation, boosting cognitive function, and lowering oxidative stress, supporting both mental clarity and physical vitality naturally.

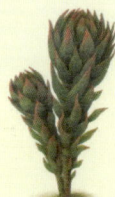

Rhodiola Rosea

Rhodiola helps improve energy and reduce fatigue by supporting the body's stress response. It enhances endurance and mental focus for sustainable energy throughout the day.

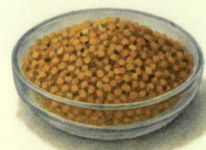

Bee Pollen

Bee pollen is rich in amino acids, vitamins, and minerals. It acts as a natural energy booster, helps combat fatigue, and supports sustained physical and mental energy throughout the day.

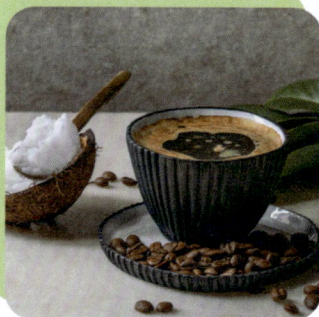

Coconut Oil Coffee Booster

Coconut oil's MCTs and coffee's caffeine offer steady energy without a crash. Cinnamon helps stabilize blood sugar for balanced focus and endurance.

Ingredients:
- 1 cup hot coffee (black or with preferred milk)
- 1 tsp coconut oil
- 1/4 tsp cinnamon

Instructions:
1. Add the coconut oil and cinnamon to hot coffee.
2. Blend or stir vigorously to create a creamy, frothy texture.
3. Sip as a morning or mid-day energy boost to power through your day.

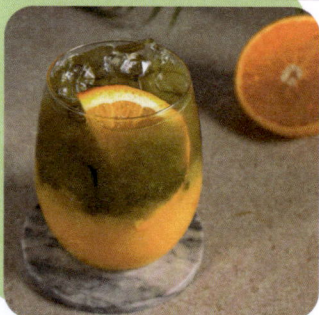

Green Tea Citrus Sparkler

Green tea's caffeine and antioxidants help fight fatigue, while orange provides natural sugars and vitamin C for a quick energy lift. This light, bubbly drink is perfect for a refreshing afternoon energy boost.

Ingredients:
- 1 cup brewed green tea, chilled
- Juice of 1/2 orange
- 1/4 cup sparkling water
- Ice cubes

Instructions:
1. Brew green tea and chill it in the refrigerator.
2. In a glass, mix chilled green tea, orange juice, and sparkling water.
3. Add ice cubes and enjoy a refreshing and energizing afternoon drink.

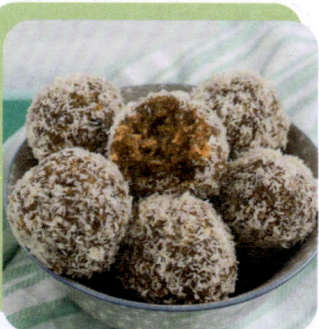

Ginger-Coconut Energy Bites

These energy bites combine coconut and ginger to provide a natural source of sustained energy. Coconut offers healthy fats for a steady energy supply, while ginger improves circulation, helping deliver nutrients more effectively.

Ingredients:
- 1/2 cup shredded coconut
- 1/4 cup rolled oats
- 1/2 tsp grated ginger
- 1 tbsp honey
- 1/2 tsp cinnamon

Instructions:
1. In a mixing bowl, combine all ingredients and mix until a dough forms.
2. Roll into small bite-sized balls and refrigerate for 15-20 minutes to set.
3. Enjoy 1-2 bites as a quick energy boost whenever needed.

Thyroid Support

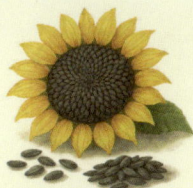

Sunflower Seeds

Sunflower seeds are rich in selenium and zinc, two essential minerals that support thyroid health and hormone production. They make an easy, nutrient-dense snack that contributes to a balanced metabolism.

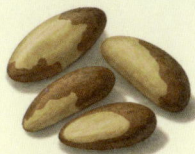

Brazil Nuts

Brazil nuts are an excellent source of selenium, a mineral essential for thyroid hormone synthesis and overall thyroid health. Just 1–2 nuts a day can help regulate metabolism, supporting proper thyroid function.

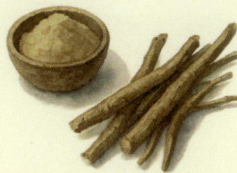

Ashwagandha

Ashwagandha supports thyroid health by balancing hormones and reducing stress. Studies have shown it can lower TSH and increase T3 and T4 levels in individuals leading to better thyroid function.

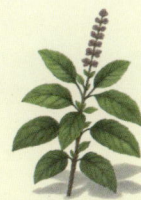

Holy Basil (Tulsi)

Holy Basil contains antioxidants and adaptogenic compounds that support the health of both the adrenal and thyroid glands. It helps balance hormone levels, reduce stress, and promote overall thyroid wellness.

Sunflower Seed & Schisandra Berry Granola

Sunflower seeds provide selenium, vitamin E, and healthy fats to support thyroid function. Schisandra berries help reduce stress and support hormone balance—making this granola a smart, metabolism-friendly choice.

Ingredients (Makes ~3 cups):

- 1½ cups rolled oats
- ½ cup raw sunflower seeds
- 2 tbsp ground flaxseed (optional, for extra fiber)
- 2 tbsp dried schisandra berries
- 1 tsp ground cinnamon
- 3 tbsp honey or maple syrup
- 2 tbsp coconut oil or olive oil

Instructions:

1. Preheat oven to 160°C (325°F) and line a baking sheet.
2. Mix oats, sunflower seeds, flaxseed, schisandra, and cinnamon in a bowl.
3. Warm honey/maple syrup and oil; pour over dry mix and stir well.
4. Spread on sheet and bake 20–25 mins, stirring halfway.
5. Cool fully, then store in an airtight jar.

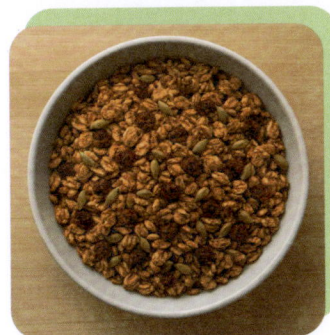

Sunflower Seed & Brazil Nut Thyroid-Boosting Pesto

This pesto blends selenium-rich Brazil nuts and zinc-packed sunflower seeds to support thyroid health. Versatile and nutrient-dense, it's perfect for salads, vegetables, or whole-grain dishes.

Ingredients:

- 1/4 cup raw sunflower seeds
- 2 Brazil nuts
- 1/2 cup fresh basil leaves (can mix with holy basil leaves if available)
- 1 clove garlic
- 1 tbsp olive oil
- Salt and pepper to taste

Instructions:

1. In a food processor, combine sunflower seeds, Brazil nuts, basil leaves, and garlic.
2. Pulse until the mixture is finely chopped.
3. Add olive oil, salt, and pepper, and process until smooth.
4. Use as a topping for salads or vegetables to add a thyroid-supportive boost to your meals.

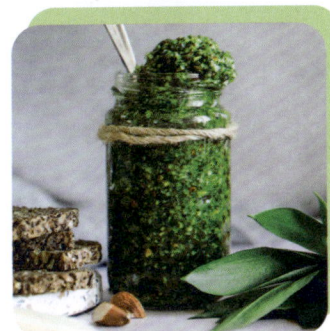

Schisandra Berry & Holy Basil Thyroid Tea

Schisandra berry is an adaptogen that supports hormonal balance, particularly in the thyroid, and helps the body adapt to stress. Holy basil (tulsi) further supports thyroid health and adrenal balance, creating a calming, supportive tea for daily use.

Ingredients:

- 1 tsp dried schisandra berries (or ½ tsp powder)
- 1 tsp dried holy basil (tulsi)
- 1 cup hot water
- ½ tsp honey or stevia (optional)

Instructions:

1. Combine schisandra berries and holy basil in a tea infuser or teapot.
2. Pour hot water over the herbs and steep for 5-7 minutes.
3. Strain, add honey if desired, and enjoy as a calming, thyroid-supportive tea once daily.

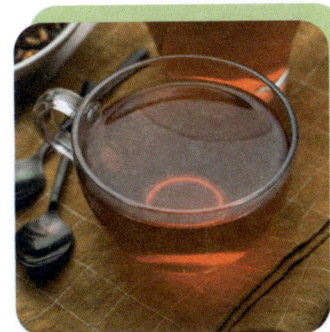

Digestive Health

Nurture your gut – explore natural solutions for digestive health, improving absorption and supporting overall gut function.

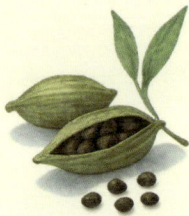

Cardamom

Cardamom helps relieve bloating, gas, and stomach cramps by relaxing digestive muscles and reducing spasms. It also supports smoother bowel movements and eases indigestion by gently stimulating gut activity when needed for improved digestive comfort.

- 1–2 grams of ground cardamom daily, or 1–2 cups of cardamom tea to support digestive health.

- One study found cardamom stimulates and relaxes gut muscles, easing constipation, cramps, and diarrhea.[85]

- Lightly dry-roast and grind the seeds just before use to release their full flavor and maximize health benefits.

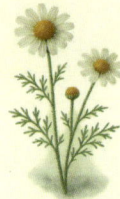

Chamomile

Chamomile contains apigenin, a compound known for its calming effects on the digestive system. It relaxes intestinal muscles, relieving cramping, bloating, and indigestion. Chamomile also has mild antibacterial properties, which help maintain gut balance.

- Brew a chamomile tea by steeping 1-2 teaspoons of dried flowers in hot water, drink 1-2 cups daily.

- A trial found chamomile tea relieved colic in 57% of infants, versus 26% with placebo.[86]

- Drink chamomile tea after meals to support digestion and help reduce post-meal bloating and discomfort.

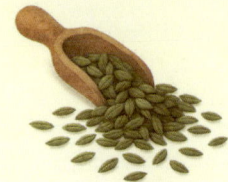

Fennel

Fennel seeds contain anethole, a compound that relaxes stomach muscles, reducing cramps and bloating. It acts as a natural carminative, helping to release trapped gas in the intestines. Fennel also has mild antimicrobial properties to support a healthy gut balance.

- Chew on 1 teaspoon of fennel seeds after meals or brew in tea for soothing effects.

- A study found fennel and turmeric extracts reduced IBS symptoms like pain and bloating in 76% of participants.[87]

- Lightly toast fennel seeds before chewing to enhance their flavor and boost their digestive benefits.

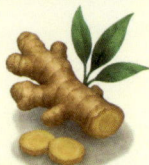

Ginger

Ginger contains gingerols and shogaols, compounds that help speed up stomach emptying and reduce bloating. They also have powerful anti-inflammatory and antioxidant effects, calming the digestive tract and helping alleviate nausea, indigestion, and overall digestive discomfort.

- Drink ginger tea made with 1-2 slices of ginger in hot water, or take 1/4 tsp of ginger powder before meals.

- Research indicates that ginger accelerates gastric emptying by 25%, enhancing digestion and reducing discomfort.[88]

- Combine ginger with a pinch of black pepper to boost its absorption and enhance its digestive benefits and overall effectiveness.

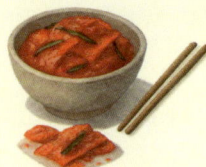

Kimchi

Fermented vegetables like sauerkraut, kimchi, and pickled beets aid digestion by providing probiotics—beneficial bacteria that help balance the gut microbiome, enhance nutrient absorption, support regular bowel movements, and strengthen the immune system through improved gut health.

- Include 1–2 tablespoons of kimchi as a side dish with meals.

- Daily kimchi improved IBS symptoms by reducing bloating, discomfort, gut inflammation, and harmful enzymes.[89]

- Choose refrigerated, unpasteurized versions to ensure you get live, active cultures that support gut health.

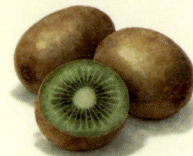

Kiwi

Kiwis are rich in fiber and contain the enzyme actinidin, which helps break down protein and speed up digestion. They also draw water into the intestines, softening stool and easing bowel movements, making them especially helpful for relieving occasional constipation and supporting overall digestive health.

- Eat 1–2 kiwis each morning (about 150–200 g total).

- Eating 2 green kiwis daily eased IBS and constipation, boosting bowel movements by 1.5+ per week and reducing bloating.[90]

- The skins are edible—just be sure to wash them well—as they provide extra fiber that supports better digestion and overall gut health.

Nurture your gut – explore natural solutions for digestive health, improving absorption and supporting overall gut function.

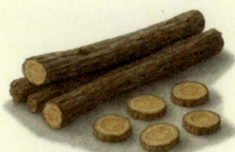

Licorice Root

Licorice root contains glycyrrhizin, a compound that helps protect the stomach lining and supports mucosal defenses, easing inflammation and pain from ulcers. It also promotes mucus production, which is highly beneficial for those with digestive distress and discomfort.

- Take 1-2 teaspoons of licorice root tea daily. Use deglycyrrhizinated licorice if taken long-term to avoid side effects.

- Licorice extract with standard treatment raised *H. pylori* clearance to 83%, compared to 62% with standard treatment alone.[91]

- Pair with ginger to amplify anti-inflammatory effects and relieve stomach discomfort.

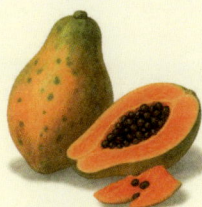

Papaya

Papaya contains papain, a natural enzyme that helps break down proteins, making it effective for improving digestion and reducing bloating. Its high fiber content also promotes regular bowel movements, making it especially beneficial for relieving constipation and supporting gut health.

- Consume 1/2 cup of fresh papaya daily, especially after meals for best results.

- A small papaya provides about 3 g of fiber, which supports regular bowel movements and overall digestive health.[92]

- Choose ripe papayas for more enzymes; blend with pineapple for a potent enzyme-rich smoothie.

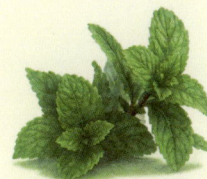

Peppermint

Peppermint contains menthol, a compound that relaxes the muscles of the gastrointestinal tract, helping to reduce bloating, cramping, and discomfort. It's widely studied for its effectiveness in soothing symptoms of IBS and supporting smoother, more comfortable digestion.

- Drink 1-2 cups of peppermint tea per day, or take enteric-coated peppermint capsules for IBS relief.

- Peppermint oil reduced IBS abdominal pain, with a 78% higher chance of relief (RR 1.78).[93]

- Avoid combining peppermint with antacids, as it can worsen acid reflux by relaxing the esophageal sphincter.

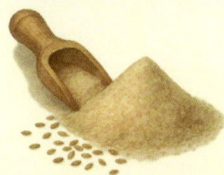

Psyllium Husk

Psyllium husk is a soluble fiber that absorbs water in the gut, forming a gel-like substance that eases stool passage and promotes regularity. In addition to relieving constipation, it acts as a prebiotic—nourishing beneficial gut bacteria and supporting a balanced, healthy microbiome for optimal digestive health.

- Start with 1 teaspoon in water daily and increase as needed, with plenty of fluids.

- A study found 7 days of psyllium improved stool consistency and frequency in constipated patients.[94]

- Mix psyllium with warm water for a smoother texture, and always avoid taking it dry to prevent choking or discomfort.

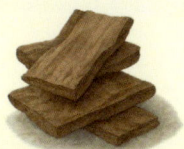

Slippery Elm

Slippery elm contains mucilage, a soothing substance that coats the digestive tract, providing relief from heartburn, acid reflux, and inflammatory bowel conditions. It forms a protective layer along the gut lining, promoting healing, reducing irritation, and enhancing overall digestive comfort and resilience.

- Mix 1 teaspoon of slippery elm powder in water and drink twice daily, preferably before meals.

- A slippery elm formula increased bowel movements by 20% and reduced straining, pain, and bloating.[95]

- Combine with marshmallow root for a potent gut-soothing blend; mix with applesauce for easy consumption.

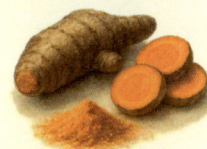

Turmeric

Turmeric contains curcumin, a powerful anti-inflammatory and antioxidant that helps reduce inflammation in the digestive tract and supports a healthy microbiome. It has shown promise in relieving symptoms of IBS and easing discomfort linked to various inflammatory digestive conditions, promoting overall gut health.

- Add 1/2-1 teaspoon of turmeric powder to meals daily.

- In 116 people with functional dyspepsia, 500 mg curcumin four times daily for 7 days improved symptoms by 60%.[96]

- Add turmeric to a smoothie with ginger and coconut oil for better absorption and enhanced anti-inflammatory effects.

Gut Health & Microbiome Support

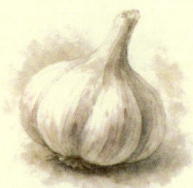

Garlic

Garlic contains allicin and prebiotics that support the growth of beneficial gut bacteria. It also acts as a natural antimicrobial, helping balance and protect gut flora effectively and naturally.

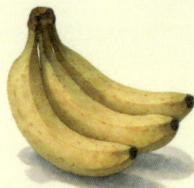

Bananas

Bananas are rich in natural fibers that feed beneficial bacteria and promote a healthy microbiome. They support digestive regularity, enhance gut balance, and contribute to overall digestive wellness.

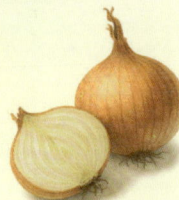

Onions

Onions are high in prebiotics like inulin and fructooligosaccharides. These compounds nourish good bacteria and help maintain a balanced, resilient gut environment.

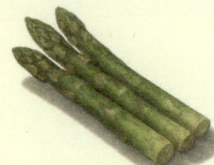

Asparagus

Asparagus is a natural source of prebiotics that support the growth of healthy gut bacteria. It helps maintain digestive balance and promotes overall microbiome health for better gut function.

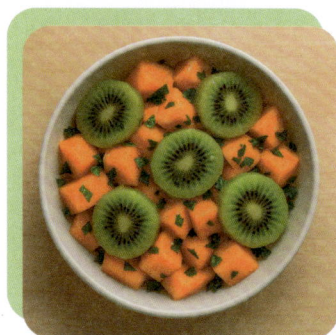

Kiwi & Papaya Citrus Salad

Kiwi and papaya offer vitamin C, antioxidants, and enzymes that aid digestion and reduce bloating. With lime and mint, this refreshing salad also supports immunity, skin health, and collagen production.

Ingredients (Serves 2):

- 2 ripe kiwis, peeled and sliced
- 1 cup ripe papaya, diced (seeds removed)
- 1 tbsp lime juice
- 1 tsp honey or maple syrup (optional, if your fruit isn't very sweet)
- Fresh mint leaves, chopped (about 1 tbsp)
- Pinch of sea salt or chili flakes (optional, for contrast)

Instructions:

1. Combine kiwi and papaya in a bowl.
2. Drizzle with lime juice and optional honey or syrup.
3. Add mint and a pinch of salt or chili flakes if desired.
4. Toss gently and let sit 5–10 mins.
5. Serve chilled as a dessert or snack.

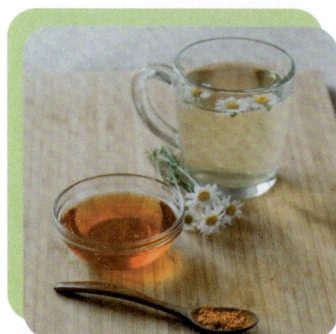

Chamomile & Turmeric Gut Tonic

This tonic combines chamomile's soothing effects with turmeric's anti-inflammatory benefits. Chamomile calms the gut lining, while turmeric reduces inflammation, supporting microbiome balance and gut health.

Ingredients:

- 1 chamomile tea bag (or 1 teaspoon dried chamomile flowers)
- 1/4 tsp turmeric powder
- 1 cup hot water
- 1 tsp apple cider vinegar (optional)

Instructions:

1. Steep chamomile in hot water for 5 minutes.
2. Remove the tea bag or strain out the flowers, then add turmeric powder and stir well.
3. Add apple cider vinegar if desired for added gut health benefits.
4. Drink warm, preferably before bedtime, to relax the gut and aid digestion.

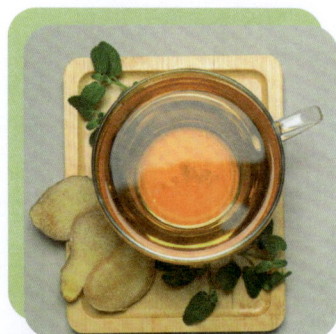

Ginger & Peppermint Gut Balancer

Ginger and peppermint work together to support gut health. Ginger stimulates digestion and reduces inflammation, while peppermint relaxes digestive muscles, easing tension and improving nutrient absorption.

Ingredients:

- 1/2 tsp grated fresh ginger (or 1/4 tsp ginger powder)
- 1 peppermint tea bag (or 1 teaspoon dried peppermint leaves)
- 1 cup hot water
- 1 tsp honey (optional)

Instructions:

1. Add ginger and peppermint to a cup, then pour hot water over them. Let steep for 5-10 minutes.
2. Remove the tea bag or strain, and add honey if desired.
3. Sip slowly, especially after meals, to help relax the gut and promote smoother digestion.

Bloating & Indigestion

EXTRA HERBS

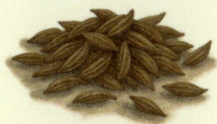

Caraway Seeds
Caraway seeds have carminative properties that help relieve bloating, gas, and indigestion. They've been traditionally used to promote digestive comfort and ease discomfort.

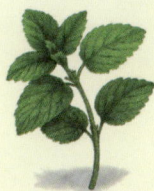

Lemon Balm
Lemon balm calms the muscles of the digestive tract, helping to reduce gas, bloating, and mild cramping. It is commonly used to support smooth, comfortable digestion and overall digestive wellness.

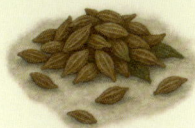

Anise
Anise contains anethole, a natural compound that relaxes digestive muscles. It helps reduce bloating, gas, and abdominal tension following meals, promoting greater digestive comfort.

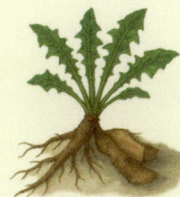

Dandelion Root
Dandelion root stimulates bile production, supporting digestion and reducing symptoms of bloating and indigestion. It also helps the body process fats more efficiently.

Fennel & Ginger Anti-Bloat Tea

This tea combines fennel seeds, known for their carminative properties to relieve gas, with ginger, which aids in digestion and reduces bloating. Together, they make a potent remedy for soothing indigestion and easing bloating.

Ingredients:
- 1 tsp fennel seeds
- 1/2 tsp freshly grated ginger (or 1/4 tsp ginger powder)
- 1 cup hot water
- 1 tsp honey (optional)

Instructions:
1. Add fennel seeds and ginger to a cup of hot water and let steep for 5-7 minutes.
2. Strain and add honey if desired.
3. Drink after meals to relieve bloating and promote better digestion.

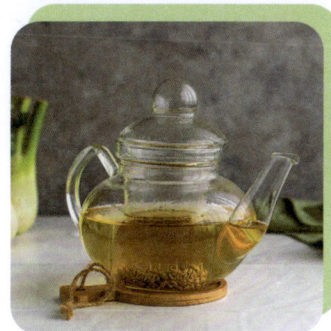

Apple Cider Vinegar & Lemon Digestive Shot

Apple cider vinegar (ACV) helps stimulate digestive enzymes and balances stomach acid, while lemon provides vitamin C and boosts digestion. This quick shot aids in reducing bloating and relieving indigestion.

Ingredients:
- 1 tbsp apple cider vinegar
- Juice of 1/2 lemon
- 1/4 cup water
- A pinch of cinnamon (optional, to enhance flavor and boost digestion)

Instructions:
1. Mix apple cider vinegar, lemon juice, and water in a small glass.
2. Add a pinch of cinnamon for taste, if desired.
3. Take this shot 10-15 minutes before meals to support digestion and reduce bloating.

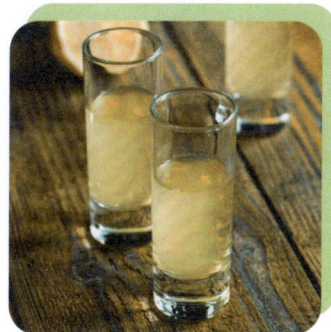

Peppermint & Chamomile Bloat Relief Infusion

Peppermint relaxes the muscles in the digestive tract, easing gas and bloating, while chamomile reduces inflammation and soothes the stomach. Together, they create a calming infusion to relieve discomfort.

Ingredients:
- 1 peppermint tea bag (or 1 tsp dried peppermint leaves)
- 1 chamomile tea bag (or 1 tsp dried chamomile flowers)
- 1 cup hot water

Instructions:
1. Place both tea bags (or loose herbs) in a cup and pour hot water over them.
2. Let steep for 5-10 minutes, then remove the tea bags or strain.
3. Drink warm after meals to help ease indigestion and bloating.

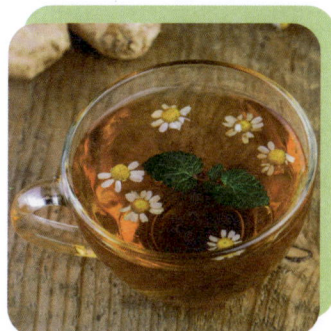

Constipation & Diarrhea

EXTRA HERBS

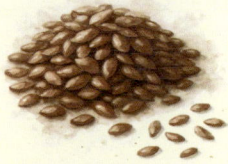

Flaxseeds

Flaxseeds are high in soluble fiber, which adds bulk to the stool and promotes regular bowel movements. They help relieve constipation, support overall gut health, and contribute to a balanced digestive system.

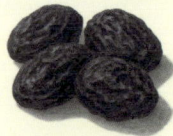

Prunes

Prunes contain both fiber and sorbitol, a natural sugar alcohol that acts as a gentle laxative. Together, these components support regular bowel movements and help ease constipation effectively.

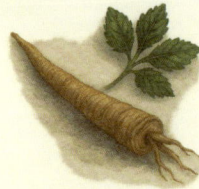

Marshmallow Root

Marshmallow root's mucilage content soothes the digestive tract and reduces inflammation. It helps manage both constipation and diarrhea by calming the gut lining.

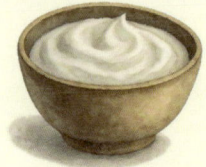

Yogurt

Yogurt provides probiotics that balance gut bacteria and support healthy digestion. Regular consumption can help ease both constipation and diarrhea by restoring microbial harmony in the gut.

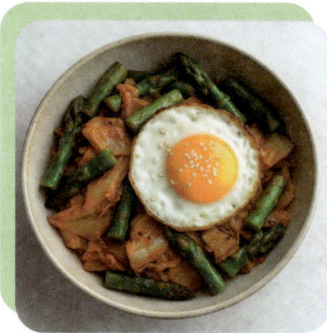

Kimchi & Asparagus Stir-Fry

Kimchi provides probiotics for gut health and immunity, while asparagus offers prebiotic fiber to feed good bacteria and support digestion—making this a powerful, gut-friendly combo.

Ingredients (Serves 2):

- 1 cup chopped kimchi
- 1 bunch asparagus, cut into 2-inch pieces
- 1 tbsp sesame or olive oil
- 2 garlic cloves, minced
- 1 tsp grated ginger (optional)
- 1 tsp soy sauce or tamari
- ½ tsp sesame seeds (optional)
- 1 soft-boiled/fried egg (optional)
- Brown rice or quinoa (optional for serving)

Instructions:

1. Heat oil in a skillet; sauté garlic (and ginger) for 30 seconds.
2. Add asparagus; cook 3–4 mins until tender-crisp.
3. Stir in kimchi and soy sauce; cook 1–2 mins more.
4. Serve over rice or quinoa, topped with sesame seeds and egg if desired.

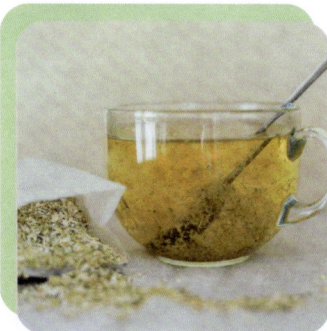

Chamomile & Psyllium Husk Digestive Drink for Regularity

Chamomile helps soothe the digestive tract, while psyllium husk provides fiber to promote regularity. This drink can aid in alleviating constipation and regulating bowel movements.

Ingredients:

- 1 chamomile tea bag (or 1 tsp dried chamomile flowers)
- 1 tsp psyllium husk powder
- 1 cup warm water
- 1 tsp honey (optional)

Instructions:

1. Steep chamomile tea bag in warm water for 5 minutes, then remove the tea bag.
2. Stir in the psyllium husk and allow it to thicken slightly.
3. Add honey if desired and drink immediately. This drink is best consumed in the evening to promote morning regularity.

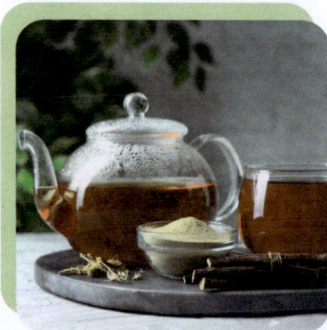

Ginger & Licorice Root Soothing Tea for Diarrhea

Ginger is known to reduce inflammation and soothe the digestive system, while licorice root helps calm the gut lining. Together, they create a gentle tea that helps reduce symptoms of diarrhea.

Ingredients:

- 1/2 tsp grated fresh ginger (or 1/4 tsp ginger powder)
- 1/2 tsp dried licorice root (or 1 licorice tea bag)
- 1 cup hot water

Instructions:

1. Add ginger and licorice root to a cup, then pour hot water over them.
2. Let steep for 10 minutes, then strain and sip slowly.
3. Drink as needed to help reduce diarrhea and soothe the digestive tract.

IBS & Other Digestive Disorders

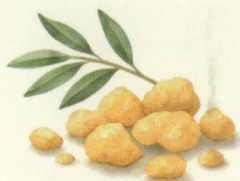

Boswellia

Boswellia contains powerful anti-inflammatory compounds that may help soothe the gut lining, making it beneficial for managing symptoms of IBS and enhancing overall gut comfort and digestive health.

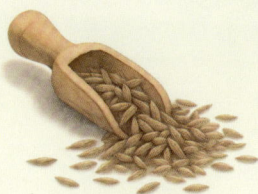

Cumin

Cumin has been shown to reduce common IBS symptoms such as bloating and abdominal pain. It aids digestion, helps minimize gas, and alleviates intestinal discomfort for improved digestive comfort.

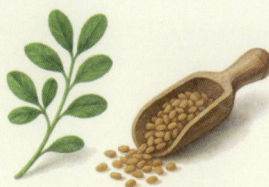

Fenugreek

Fenugreek is rich in mucilage, a soothing compound that helps calm inflammation in the digestive tract. It may also help alleviate discomfort and support digestive health in individuals with IBS.

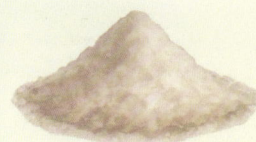

L-Glutamine

L-Glutamine is an amino acid that supports the repair of the gut lining. It promotes digestive health and may help reduce symptoms of IBS by strengthening intestinal integrity and the gut barrier function.

Slippery Elm & Chamomile Calming Digestive Drink

Slippery elm forms a soothing gel that coats the digestive tract, providing relief from irritation and inflammation, while chamomile further calms the stomach and helps manage IBS-related discomfort.

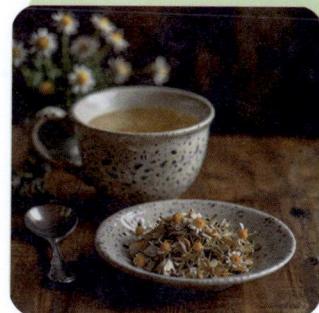

Ingredients:
- 1 tsp slippery elm powder
- 1 chamomile tea bag (or 1 teaspoon dried chamomile flowers)
- 1 cup warm water

Instructions:
1. Steep chamomile in warm water for 5 minutes, then remove the tea bag.
2. Stir in slippery elm powder until fully dissolved.
3. Drink once daily to help soothe the digestive tract and alleviate IBS symptoms.

Cardamom & Prune Digestive Energy Balls

These energy balls blend cardamom for digestion, prunes for gentle relief and gut motility, and nuts/seeds for lasting energy—making them a gut-friendly, blood sugar–stable snack.

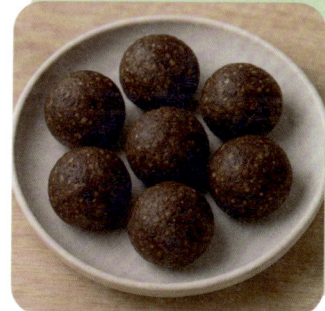

Ingredients (Makes ~12 balls):
- ½ cup pitted Medjool dates
- ¼ cup prunes
- ½ cup almonds or cashews
- 2 tbsp sunflower or pumpkin seeds
- 1 tbsp chia seeds (optional)
- ½ tsp cardamom
- ¼ tsp cinnamon
- Pinch of sea salt
- 1 tsp coconut oil (if needed)

Instructions:
1. Pulse nuts and seeds in a food processor.
2. Add remaining ingredients and blend into a sticky dough.
3. Roll into small balls.
Optional: Coat with coconut or sesame
4. seeds.
5. Store in the fridge for 1 week or freeze for longer.

Fenugreek & L-Glutamine Gut Repair Smoothie

Fenugreek helps reduce inflammation and supports gut health, while L-glutamine is an amino acid that plays a vital role in maintaining the gut lining, making this smoothie beneficial for soothing and repairing the digestive tract, especially during IBS flare-ups.

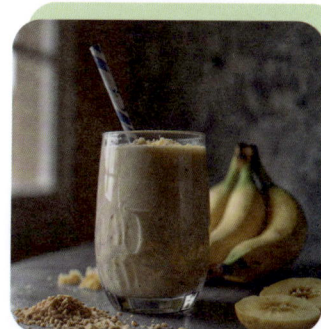

Ingredients:
- 1 tsp soaked fenugreek seeds or ¼ tsp powder
- ½ tsp L-glutamine powder
- ½ cup coconut water or almond milk
- ½ banana

Instructions:
1. Add soaked fenugreek seeds (or fenugreek powder), L-glutamine powder, coconut water, and banana to a blender.
2. Blend until smooth.
3. Drink in the morning to soothe the gut, reduce inflammation, and support a healthy digestive tract.

Hair & Nail Health

Achieve strong, vibrant hair and nails – discover foods and herbs that promote growth, strength, and vitality from within.

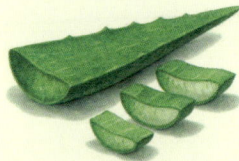

Aloe Vera

Aloe vera contains proteolytic enzymes that help repair scalp skin and moisturize hair. Its antibacterial and antifungal properties support a healthy scalp environment. For nails, its hydrating effects combined with vitamin E help prevent brittleness and promote stronger, healthier growth.

- Massage fresh aloe gel into the scalp for 5 mins, then rinse after 30. For nails, apply a thin layer and leave overnight.

- Using 0.5% Aloe vera cream three times daily for four weeks cured 83% of mild to moderate psoriasis cases.[97]

- Refrigerate the gel before application to enhance its cooling, soothing, and potent anti-inflammatory effect naturally.

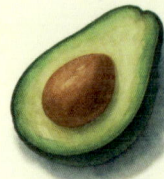

Avocado

Avocado is rich in essential fatty acids and vitamins E and B, which nourish hair by restoring shine, sealing in moisture, and reducing damage. Its high vitamin E content also strengthens nails, reduces splitting, and promotes healthy growth and resilience.

- Apply mashed avocado to damp hair for 20 minutes, then rinse. Rub a small amount on nails and cuticles daily.

- Eating 1 avocado daily for eight weeks improved skin elasticity and firmness in healthy women.[98]

- Mix with a teaspoon of olive oil for added hydration, deeply enhancing both scalp and hair health and shine.

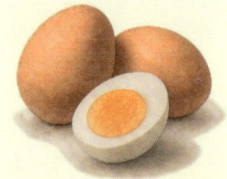

Biotin-Rich Foods

Eggs are a powerhouse of biotin, a B vitamin essential for producing keratin—the main protein in hair and nails. This nutrient helps reduce breakage, supports healthy hair growth, and naturally improves nail strength, thickness, and resilience.

- Eat 1–2 eggs daily for biotin and protein. Use in hair masks for extra nourishment.

- Eating a cooked egg supplies 10 micrograms of biotin, covering one-third of your daily requirement.[99]

- Combine with foods high in zinc, like pumpkin seeds, for maximum keratin production and stronger hair growth.

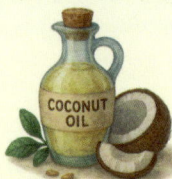

Coconut Oil

Coconut oil penetrates deep into hair shafts, providing intense hydration and minimizing protein loss, which is vital for reducing breakage and maintaining strong, healthy hair. Its nourishing fatty acids also benefit nails by moisturizing cuticles and helping reduce nail splitting, brittleness, and damage.

- Massage 1 tsp of coconut oil into the scalp or hair; leave for 1 hour or overnight. Rub a small amount on cuticles daily.

- Coconut oil before and after washing can cut protein loss by up to 39%, to strengthen hair and prevent damage.[100]

- Warm the oil slightly before applying to enhance absorption and achieve deeper hydration and nourishment.

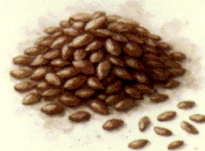

Flaxseeds

Flaxseeds contain high levels of omega-3 fatty acids, which deeply nourish hair follicles and promote elasticity, naturally reducing breakage and enhancing shine for healthier, more vibrant hair. They also strengthen nails by reducing brittleness and encouraging smooth, fast, healthy, and resilient growth over time.

- Consume 1–2 tablespoons of ground flaxseeds daily in smoothies or yogurt.

- Omega-3s have been shown to improve hair elasticity by up to 30%.[101]

- Grind fresh flaxseeds as needed to retain omega-3 potency, as whole seeds can pass undigested and reduce nutrient absorption.

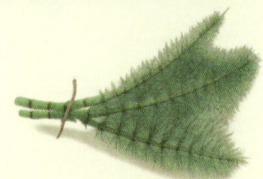

Horsetail

Horsetail is rich in silica, a mineral essential for collagen production that supports the structure and strength of both hair and nails. It helps strengthen weak, brittle hair and nails while promoting faster, healthier, and more resilient growth for improved overall vitality, appearance, texture, and shine.

- Drink 1 cup of horsetail tea daily or use as a weekly hair rinse. Soak nails in cooled tea for 5–10 minutes.

- Daily horsetail-derived silica supplements boosted hair growth in women with thinning hair over 90–180 days.[102]

- Combine with nettle or rosemary tea to boost scalp circulation and support healthy, vigorous, and sustained hair growth.

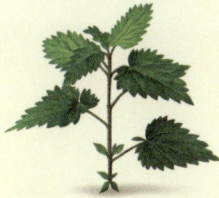

Hair & Nail Health

Nettle Leaf

Nettle leaf is rich in vitamins A, C, D, and K, along with essential minerals like iron and silica, which promote hair growth by improving blood flow to the scalp. Its natural anti-inflammatory properties also help reduce scalp irritation and support overall scalp health.

- Steep 1–2 teaspoons of dried nettle for tea, or take a 500 mg capsule daily.

- Applying nettle leaf extract topically can boost hair growth by 10% in six months.[103]

- Combine nettle tea with rosemary for an extra boost in hair growth, scalp health, overall hair vitality, and strength.

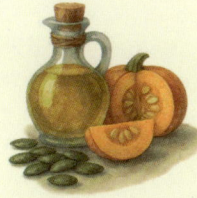

Pumpkin Seed Oil

Pumpkin seed oil is rich in zinc and essential fatty acids that nourish hair follicles, strengthen nail beds, and enhance overall scalp health. Its phytosterols help inhibit enzymes associated with hair loss, making it effective for promoting fuller, stronger hair growth.

- Take 1-2 teaspoons of pumpkin seed oil daily or add to salads and smoothies.

- Taking 400 mg of pumpkin seed oil daily can boost hair count by 40% in 24 weeks.[104]

- Look for cold-pressed pumpkin seed oil for the highest concentration of beneficial nutrients and natural antioxidants.

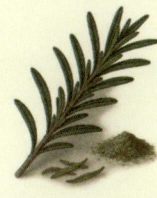

Rosemary

Rosemary contains ursolic acid, which boosts circulation to hair follicles, encouraging stronger, thicker hair growth. Its antioxidant and antimicrobial properties protect the scalp from damage, making it ideal for promoting overall hair and nail health.

- Apply diluted rosemary oil to the scalp twice a week or drink rosemary tea regularly.

- Daily rosemary oil use increased hair count by 22.4% in six months, similar to 2% minoxidil.[105]

- Massage the scalp for five minutes after applying rosemary oil to further stimulate blood flow and promote hair growth.

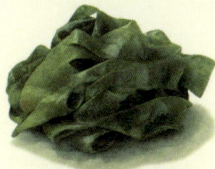

Seaweed

Seaweed is rich in essential nutrients like iodine, zinc, iron, and vitamins A and C, which support healthy growth and strength. Its high mineral content nourishes hair follicles, improves scalp circulation, and strengthens brittle nails for overall hair and nail health, vitality, natural beauty, and resilience.

- 1–2 servings per week (about 5–10 grams dried or a handful fresh) of edible seaweed.

- Grateloupia elliptica may prevent hair loss by boosting hair cell growth, blocking DHT, reducing inflammation, and fighting dandruff.[106]

- Add seaweed to soups, salads, or rice bowls—or try a seaweed face mask for a skin-boosting treat from the outside in.

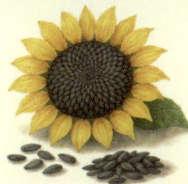

Sunflower Seeds

Sunflower seeds are rich in vitamin E and zinc, both essential for maintaining strong, healthy hair and nails. Vitamin E enhances scalp health by improving circulation, while zinc plays a crucial role in promoting hair growth and reducing shedding, supporting overall hair vitality, strength, and natural shine.

- Consume a small handful (about 1 ounce) of sunflower seeds daily as a snack or salad topping.

- Consuming vitamin E-rich foods like sunflower seeds can boost hair growth by 34.5% over eight months.[107]

- Opt for unsalted sunflower seeds to keep sodium intake low and maximize the benefits of their nutrient content.

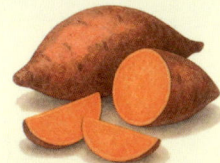

Sweet Potatoes

Sweet potatoes are a rich source of beta-carotene, which the body converts to vitamin A—an essential nutrient for cell regeneration and scalp health. This nutrient helps improve hair strength and shine, while also supporting stronger nail growth, durability, overall resilience, and healthy appearance.

- Include half a cup of roasted sweet potatoes in meals 2-3 times a week.

- Consuming a medium sweet potato daily can supply 160% of your vitamin A requirement.[108]

- Pair sweet potatoes with healthy fats (like olive oil) to enhance the absorption of beta-carotene and improve overall nutrient uptake.

Hair Growth & Strengthening

EXTRA HERBS

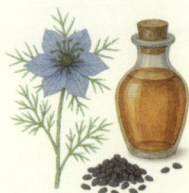

Black Seed Oil

Black seed oil contains thymoquinone, a potent antioxidant that strengthens hair follicles and helps reduce thinning, supporting healthy, fuller, thicker, and more resilient hair growth.

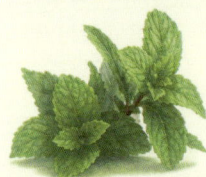

Peppermint Oil

Peppermint oil, rich in menthol, stimulates scalp circulation, which promotes hair growth and strengthens hair roots by increasing nutrient delivery to follicles, improving overall scalp health.

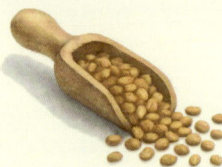

Fenugreek Seeds

Fenugreek seeds are high in protein and nicotinic acid, both of which help repair hair follicles, reduce hair loss, improve hair density over time, and promote stronger, healthier hair growth naturally.

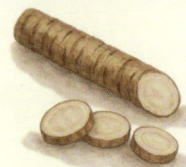

Burdock Root

Burdock root is rich in essential fatty acids and phytosterols that nourish the scalp. It supports healthy hair thickness, promotes growth, and helps maintain overall scalp and follicle health.

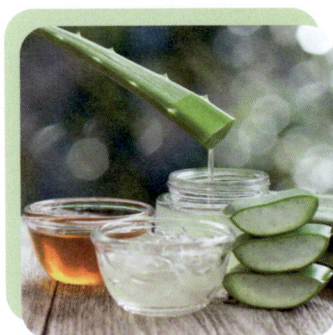

Nourishing Rosemary & Coconut Oil Scalp Treatment

Rosemary and coconut oil are celebrated for their potential to stimulate hair follicles, strengthen strands, and provide deep moisture. This duo supports scalp health, encouraging hair growth and minimizing breakage.

Ingredients:

- 2 tbsp coconut oil
- 5 drops rosemary essential oil
- 1 tbsp aloe vera gel

Instructions:

1. Warm the coconut oil slightly until it's melted (avoid making it hot).
2. Add the rosemary essential oil and aloe vera gel, mixing well.
3. Massage the mixture into your scalp, focusing on roots. Leave on for 30 minutes to 1 hour before rinsing with
4. shampoo.
5. Use once or twice a week for best results.

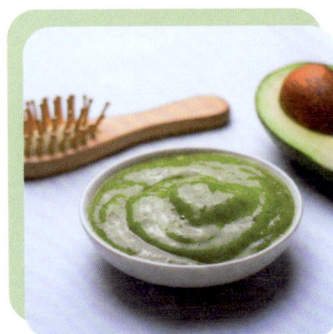

Avocado & Biotin Boost Hair Mask

This mask blends avocado, rich in vitamins and healthy fats, with biotin from eggs to support hair's protein structure, enhancing strength and shine.

Ingredients:

- 1/2 ripe avocado
- 1 egg (biotin-rich)
- 1 tbsp olive oil

Instructions:

1. Mash the avocado until smooth.
2. Whisk the egg separately, then mix it into the avocado along with olive oil.
3. Apply the mask from roots to tips, covering hair with a shower cap.
4. Let sit for 20-30 minutes, then rinse with cool water and shampoo.
5. Use weekly for improved hair strength and vitality.

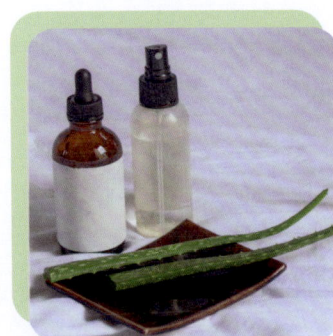

Aloe Vera & Peppermint Scalp Spray

This refreshing scalp spray uses aloe vera to soothe and hydrate, while peppermint invigorates the scalp, increasing circulation to support hair growth.

Ingredients:

- 1/2 cup aloe vera juice
- 5 drops peppermint essential oil
- 1/2 cup water

Instructions:

1. Mix aloe vera juice, water, and peppermint oil in a spray bottle.
2. Shake well and spray directly onto your scalp, massaging gently.
3. Use daily or as needed for a refreshing and growth-boosting scalp treatment.

Nail Health & Strength

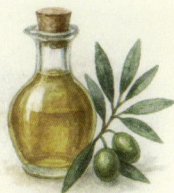

Olive Oil

Olive oil is rich in vitamin E and deeply moisturizes nails and cuticles. It helps strengthen brittle nails, improving their flexibility, durability, strength, resilience, and preventing breakage.

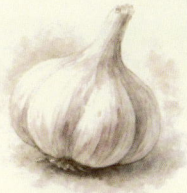

Garlic

Garlic contains selenium, a mineral that supports nail strength and growth. Applying garlic extract regularly can enhance nail hardness, thickness, and overall resilience naturally.

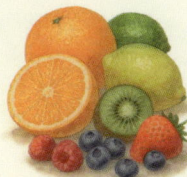

Vitamin C-Rich Foods

Vitamin C is vital for collagen production, which helps maintain strong, healthy nails. Regular intake reduces brittleness and promotes consistent nail growth.

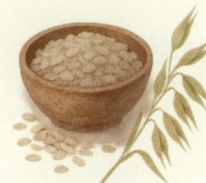

Oats

Oats are a widely available whole grain rich in bioavailable silicon (SiO_2), which supports keratin and collagen formation, strengthening hair and nails and reducing breakage significantly.

Nettle & Lemon Nail Soak

The minerals in nettle promote nail health, while lemon helps strengthen and brighten nails, leaving them looking healthy and resilient.

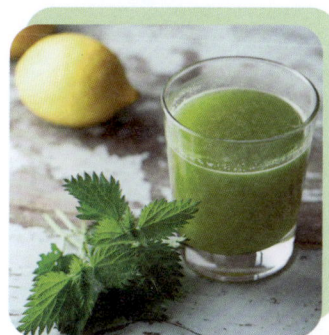

Ingredients:
- 1 tbsp dried nettle leaves
- 1 cup boiling water
- Juice of half a lemon

Instructions:
1. Steep the nettle leaves in boiling water for 10 minutes, then strain and allow to cool.
2. Add the lemon juice to the nettle tea.
3. Soak nails in the mixture for 10-15 minutes.
4. Rinse hands and apply moisturizer. Use weekly for best results.

Pumpkin Seed & Sunflower Seed Oil Nail Serum

Rich in zinc and vitamin E, this serum uses pumpkin and sunflower seed oils to nourish, strengthen, and hydrate nails.

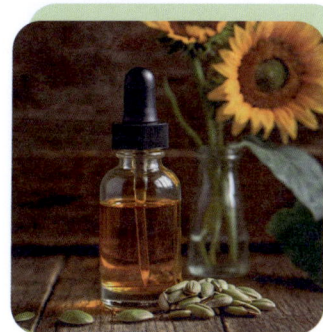

Ingredients:
- 1/2 tsp pumpkin seed oil
- 1/2 tsp sunflower seed oil

Instructions:
1. Mix the oils in a small bowl.
2. Using a cotton swab, apply the serum to nails and cuticles.
3. Massage gently and leave on overnight. Use 2-3 times per week for best results.

Flaxseed & Coconut Oil Cuticle Balm

Flaxseed oil is rich in omega-3s, helping strengthen nails and cuticles, while coconut oil provides deep hydration.

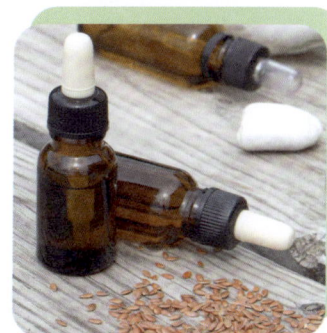

Ingredients:
- 1 tbsp flaxseed oil
- 1 tbsp coconut oil
- 3 drops lavender essential oil (optional for soothing)

Instructions:
1. Melt the coconut oil if solid, then mix with flaxseed oil and lavender oil (if using).
2. Apply to cuticles and nails, massaging gently.
3. Use nightly for soft, strong cuticles and nails.

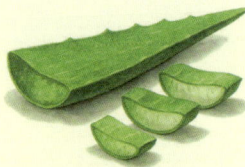

Skin Health

Aloe Vera

Aloe vera soothes irritated skin, hydrates deeply, and promotes healing with its vitamins A, C, and E. Its anti-inflammatory and antimicrobial properties help calm acne, reduce redness, support overall skin regeneration, and restore natural skin balance.

🍽 Apply fresh gel directly to skin 1–2 times daily for soothing, healing, and hydration.

⚗ Aloe vera gel speeds up the healing of second-degree burns by nearly four days.[109]

🌿 Use pure gel to soothe burns, reduce redness, and hydrate irritated or acne-prone skin, promoting healing and comfort.

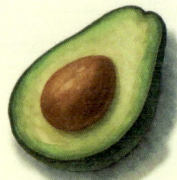

Avocado

Avocado is rich in healthy fats, vitamin E, and antioxidants that nourish and moisturize the skin. It helps improve elasticity, calm inflammation, protect against oxidative damage, and promote a softer, smoother, and more resilient complexion.

🍽 Apply mashed avocado as a face mask 2–3 times weekly; leave on for 15–20 minutes.

⚗ Eating an avocado each day for two months enhances skin elasticity and firmness.[110]

🌿 Apply as a moisturizing mask to nourish dry skin and improve elasticity with healthy fats, vitamins, and antioxidants.

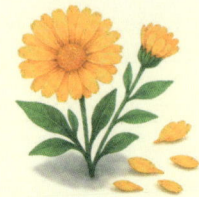

Calendula

Calendula contains flavonoids and triterpenoids that promote wound healing, reduce inflammation, and soothe irritated or sensitive skin. Its gentle antimicrobial properties make it ideal for calming eczema, acne, rashes, sunburn, and minor skin injuries.

🍽 Use calendula cream or oil 1–2 times daily on irritated or sensitive skin.

⚗ Using a 2% Calendula extract on hand wounds accelerates healing by nearly five days.[111]

🌿 Use calendula cream to calm sensitive skin, reduce inflammation, and support wound healing.

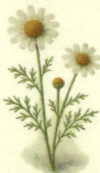

Chamomile

Chamomile is rich in antioxidants and anti-inflammatory compounds that help soothe sensitive or irritated skin. It reduces redness, calms eczema and rosacea, and protects the skin from environmental stress. It also promotes healing, supports skin renewal and hydration, and enhances softness and overall radiance.

🍽 Apply cooled chamomile tea as a toner or compress once daily; or use diluted essential oil.

⚗ Chamomile extract sped up wound healing, cutting recovery time by about 4.6 days.[112]

🌿 Apply chamomile tea or extract to relieve redness, soothe eczema, and gently calm sensitive skin, promoting healing and reducing irritation.

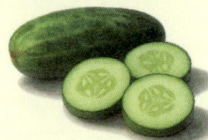

Cucumber

Cucumber hydrates and cools the skin with its high water content. It contains antioxidants and silica that reduce puffiness, calm irritation, tighten pores, and promote a refreshed, soothed, radiant, naturally glowing, healthier-looking, revitalized, and balanced complexion.

🍽 Place fresh cucumber slices on skin for 10–15 minutes daily; or blend and apply juice.

⚗ Using a 3% cucumber extract cream can lighten skin by reducing melanin levels.[113]

🌿 Use slices or juice to reduce puffiness, tighten pores, and hydrate skin naturally for a refreshed, glowing, and balanced complexion.

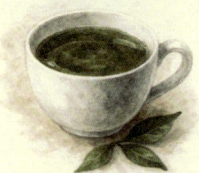

Green Tea

Green tea is rich in polyphenols like EGCG, which fight inflammation and protect the skin from UV damage. It helps reduce acne, soothe inflammation, prevent premature aging, and support clear, balanced, healthy-looking, radiant, naturally rejuvenated, and glowing skin.

🍽 Apply cooled green tea topically once daily; or use green tea extract in creams.

⚗ 2% green tea lotion twice daily for six weeks can reduce acne lesions by 58%.[114]

🌿 Mix matcha powder with yogurt for an antioxidant-rich acne mask—calms inflammation and tightens pores.

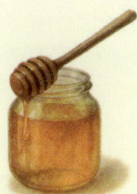

Glow from within – explore natural remedies that rejuvenate skin, reduce inflammation, and promote a clear, healthy complexion.

Honey

Honey is a natural humectant that draws moisture into the skin. With antibacterial and healing properties, it helps treat acne and supports the skin barrier, promoting soft, hydrated, radiant, glowing, visibly healthier, and more balanced skin.

- Apply raw honey directly to skin 2–3 times weekly; leave on for 15–20 minutes.

- Using honey on partial-thickness burns speeds up healing by nearly five days.[115]

- Dab on pimples overnight to reduce size and redness—also speeds healing of scabs without scarring.

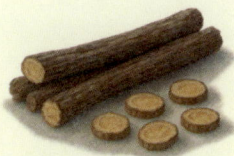

Licorice Root

Licorice root brightens skin by reducing hyperpigmentation and calming inflammation. It contains glabridin, which soothes redness, fights free radicals, and helps treat conditions like melasma, eczema, uneven skin tone, and sun-induced discoloration.

- Use creams containing 1–2% licorice extract once or twice daily for brightening or soothing.

- Using a 2% licorice root extract gel twice daily for two weeks reduces melasma pigmentation by over 15%.[116]

- Use consistently in a serum to fade melasma and PIH (post-inflammatory hyperpigmentation)— excellent after acne or sun damage.

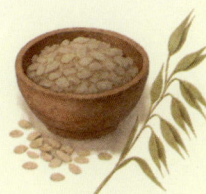

Oats

Oats are rich in beta-glucan and avenanthramides, which moisturize, soothe irritation, and reduce itching. Ideal for sensitive or eczema-prone skin, they help strengthen the skin barrier, relieve inflammation, and support overall skin health and comfort.

- Apply colloidal oatmeal paste or soak 2–3 times weekly for 15–20 minutes to soothe skin.

- 1% colloidal oatmeal cream twice daily for two weeks reduced mild to moderate dermatitis symptoms by 61%.[117]

- Make a DIY oat-milk cleanser to calm flare-ups—perfect during eczema or psoriasis outbreaks.

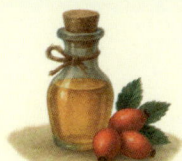

Rosehip Oil

Rosehip oil is high in vitamins A and C, which support collagen production and skin regeneration. Its fatty acids deeply hydrate, fade scars and dark spots, improve skin tone and texture, and promote a smoother, brighter, youthful, healthier-looking, and more even complexion.

- Massage a few drops into clean skin once daily, preferably at night.

- Using rosehip oil twice daily for 12 weeks reduces post-surgical scar discoloration in 63% of users.[118]

- Apply with a jade roller at night to boost circulation and fade acne scars more effectively for smoother, clearer, radiant skin.

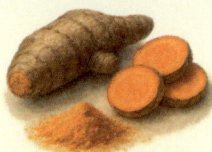

Turmeric

Turmeric contains curcumin, a powerful anti-inflammatory and antioxidant compound. It helps reduce acne, brighten the skin, fade hyperpigmentation, and protect against environmental damage while supporting an even, radiant, healthy, glowing, vibrant, and nourished complexion.

- Mix turmeric with yogurt or honey; apply mask 1–2 times weekly for 10–15 minutes.

- Turmeric extract cream application twice daily for nine weeks can reduce psoriasis severity by over 58%.[119]

- Mix with milk and chickpea flour for a brightening mask that also helps with ingrown hairs and dullness.

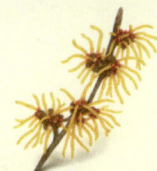

Witch Hazel

Witch hazel is a natural astringent with anti-inflammatory and antimicrobial properties. It helps tighten pores, reduce excess oil, calm acne and irritation, and tone the skin without over-drying or stripping moisture, leaving it clear, balanced, refreshed, soothed, visibly healthier, and more refined.

- Apply alcohol-free witch hazel toner once daily with a cotton pad after cleansing.

- Witch hazel extract cream used twice daily for four weeks enhances eyelid dermatitis symptoms.[120]

- Use after shaving or waxing to prevent razor bumps and soothe irritation—opt for alcohol-free formulas to avoid dryness.

Acne & Blemishes

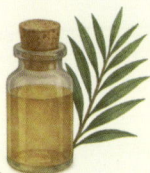

Tea Tree Oil

Tea tree oil contains terpinen-4-ol, a compound with strong antibacterial and anti-inflammatory properties. It helps reduce acne by targeting bacteria and calming skin irritation.

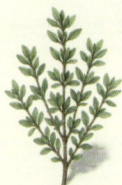

Thyme

Thyme is known for its potent antimicrobial effects. Extracts from thyme have been shown to reduce acne by eliminating bacteria that contribute to breakouts, and supporting clearer, healthier skin.

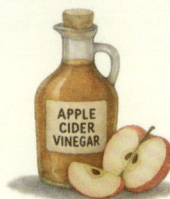

Apple Cider Vinegar

Apple cider vinegar contains acetic acid and alpha-hydroxy acids that exfoliate skin, kill bacteria, and balance pH—helping to clear blemishes and reduce acne flare-ups.

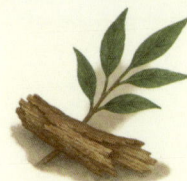

Willow Bark

Willow bark is a natural source of salicylic acid. It helps exfoliate dead skin cells, unclog pores, and reduce breakouts by supporting healthy skin turnover and promoting a clearer, smoother complexion.

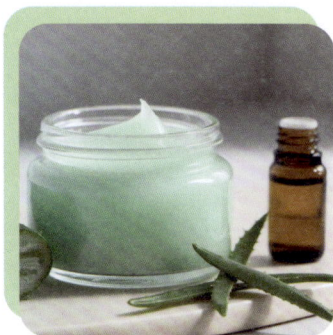

Aloe & Tea Tree Blemish Spot Treatment

Aloe Vera soothes and hydrates inflamed skin, while tea tree oil offers antibacterial properties that help combat acne-causing bacteria.

Ingredients:
- 1 tbsp Aloe Vera gel
- 2-3 drops Tea Tree oil

Instructions:
1. Mix Aloe Vera gel with tea tree oil until well combined.
2. Apply a thin layer to acne-prone areas or spots.
3. Leave on for 15-20 minutes, then rinse with lukewarm water. Use 1-2 times daily as needed.

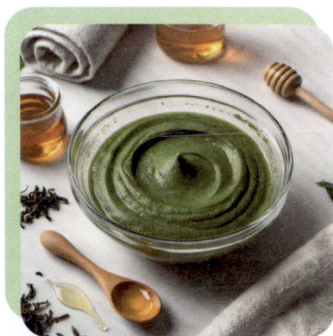

Green Tea & Honey Clarifying Mask

Green tea contains antioxidants and anti-inflammatory catechins that help reduce acne, while honey adds hydration and acts as a natural antibacterial.

Ingredients:
- 1 green tea bag (brewed, cooled, and opened to use tea leaves)
- 1 tbsp raw honey

Instructions:
1. Mix green tea leaves with honey to form a paste.
2. Apply to clean, dry skin and let sit for 10-15 minutes.
3. Rinse with warm water and pat dry. Use 2-3 times a week.

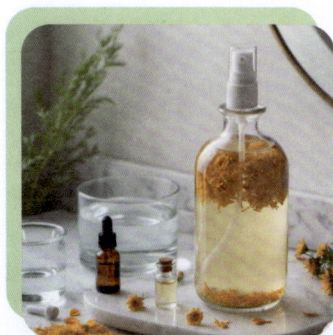

Calendula & Witch Hazel Toning Mist

Calendula reduces redness and inflammation, while witch hazel acts as a natural astringent, helping to control oil and tighten pores.

Ingredients:
- 1 cup water
- 1 tbsp dried calendula flowers
- 1 tbsp witch hazel

Instructions:
1. Steep calendula flowers in boiling water for 10 minutes, then strain and let cool.
2. Add witch hazel to the cooled calendula infusion and pour into a spray bottle.
3. Mist on face after cleansing. Store in the refrigerator for up to a week.

Skin Conditions

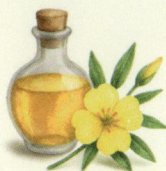

Evening Primrose Oil

Evening primrose oil contains gamma-linolenic acid (GLA), which helps reduce inflammation, dryness, and itching often associated with eczema and psoriasis.

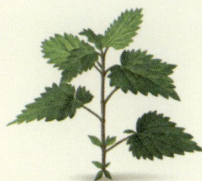

Stinging Nettle

Stinging nettle is rich in antioxidants and anti-inflammatory compounds. When used topically, it may help soothe irritation and alleviate symptoms of inflammatory skin conditions.

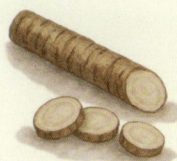

Burdock Root

Burdock root is known for its detoxifying properties. It supports skin healing, reduces redness, and can improve inflammatory skin issues like eczema, psoriasis, acne, and chronic irritation.

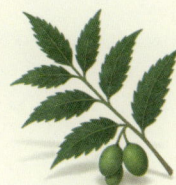

Neem

Neem contains nimbin and quercetin, which have powerful anti-inflammatory and antibacterial effects. It helps calm irritated skin and reduce eczema and psoriasis symptoms.

Oat & Honey Soothing Bath Soak

Oats are excellent for calming skin irritation, while honey adds moisture and helps reduce inflammation.

Ingredients:
- 1 cup oats (ground)
- 2 tbsp honey

Instructions:
1. Add ground oats and honey to a warm bath.
2. Soak in the bath for 15-20 minutes, gently massaging the skin as needed.
3. Rinse with lukewarm water and pat dry. Use 2-3 times a week.

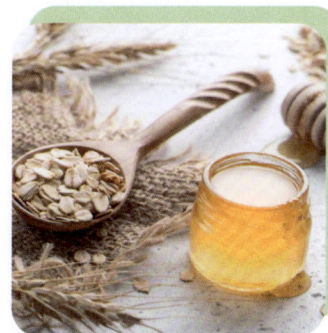

Licorice Root & Coconut Oil Calming Balm

Licorice root contains anti-inflammatory properties helpful for eczema, and coconut oil hydrates and forms a protective barrier on the skin.

Ingredients:
- 1 tsp licorice root powder
- 2 tbsp coconut oil

Instructions:
1. Mix licorice root powder into melted coconut oil until well combined.
2. Apply a thin layer to affected areas and leave on.
3. Use daily or as needed for dry, irritated skin.

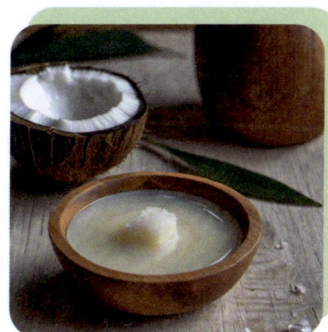

Chamomile & Aloe Vera Relief Gel

Chamomile reduces inflammation, while Aloe Vera cools and soothes irritated skin.

Ingredients:
- 1 tbsp chamomile tea (brewed and cooled)
- 1 tbsp Aloe Vera gel

Instructions:
1. Mix chamomile tea with Aloe Vera gel.
2. Apply to inflamed or itchy areas.
3. Use as a leave-on treatment daily or as needed.

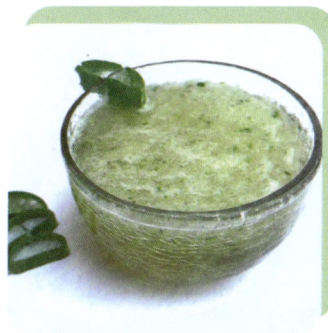

Anti-aging & Wrinkles

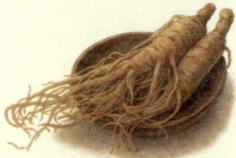

Ginseng

Ginseng is rich in antioxidants and ginsenosides that support skin regeneration. It helps reduce wrinkles, improve elasticity, and promote a smoother, more youthful appearance.

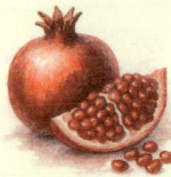

Pomegranate

Pomegranate contains ellagic acid and powerful antioxidants that protect the skin from free radical damage, reduce fine lines, boost collagen production, and enhance hydration for healthy skin.

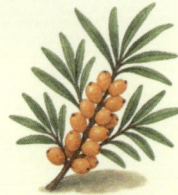

Sea Buckthorn

Sea buckthorn is high in omega-7 fatty acids, which support collagen production and skin elasticity. It helps reduce the appearance of fine lines and improve overall skin texture.

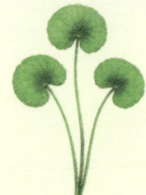

Gotu Kola

Gotu kola enhances collagen synthesis and boosts skin firmness. It's effective in preventing wrinkles, improving elasticity, and promoting a youthful, resilient, and revitalized complexion.

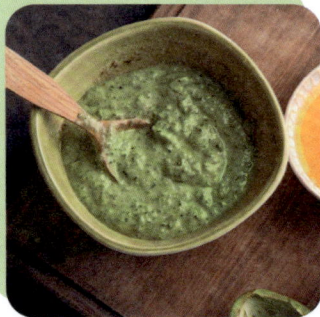

Avocado & Rosehip Nourishing Mask

Avocado provides rich hydration and antioxidants, while rosehip oil offers vitamin C and fatty acids that help improve skin elasticity.

Ingredients:
- 1/2 ripe avocado
- 5 drops rosehip oil

Instructions:
1. Mash avocado until smooth, then mix in rosehip oil.
2. Apply a thick layer to the face and neck.
3. Leave on for 15-20 minutes, then rinse off with lukewarm water. Use once a week.

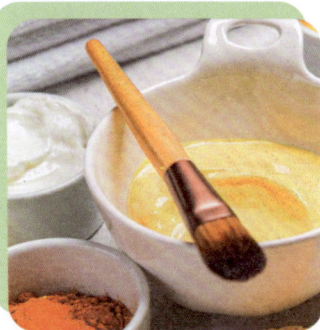

Turmeric & Yogurt Brightening Mask

Turmeric contains curcumin, a powerful antioxidant that can help reduce fine lines, while yogurt provides lactic acid for gentle exfoliation.

Ingredients:
- 1/2 tsp turmeric powder
- 1 tbsp plain yogurt

Instructions:
1. Mix turmeric with yogurt to form a smooth paste.
2. Apply to clean, dry skin and leave on for 10-15 minutes.
3. Rinse with lukewarm water. Use once a week for a radiant complexion.

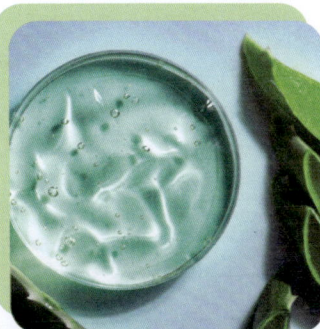

Cucumber & Green Tea Cooling Eye Gel

Cucumber's hydrating and cooling properties help reduce puffiness, while green tea provides antioxidants that help firm and refresh delicate eye areas.

Ingredients:
- 1/2 cucumber (blended)
- 1 tbsp brewed green tea (cooled)

Instructions:
1. Blend cucumber and strain the juice. Mix with green tea.
2. Apply around the eye area with a cotton pad.
3. Let sit for 10 minutes, then gently rinse. Use daily for best results.

Wound Healing & Scar Reduction

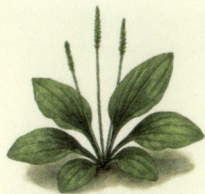

Plantain Leaf

Plantain leaf contains allantoin and antimicrobial compounds that promote cell growth, reduce inflammation, and accelerate wound healing. It also helps minimize scarring and soothes irritated skin.

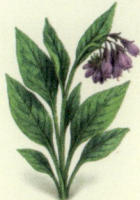

Comfrey

Comfrey is rich in allantoin, which supports rapid cell regeneration and wound healing. It helps reduce inflammation and the formation of scars during the healing process.

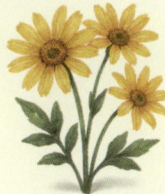

Arnica

Arnica is known for its powerful anti-inflammatory properties. It reduces bruising, swelling, and discomfort while supporting faster wound healing, minimizing scar tissue, and soothing sore skin.

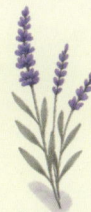

Lavender Oil

Lavender oil has antiseptic and anti-inflammatory properties that promote wound healing. It also supports skin regeneration, helps reduce scarring over time, and soothes irritation.

Gotu Kola & Honey Healing Paste

Gotu Kola supports skin repair and collagen production, while honey offers antibacterial protection to prevent infection.

Ingredients:
- 1/2 tsp Gotu Kola powder
- 1 tbsp honey

Instructions:
1. Mix Gotu Kola powder with honey to form a paste.
2. Apply to scars or healing wounds.
3. Leave on for 20-30 minutes, then rinse. Use it daily.

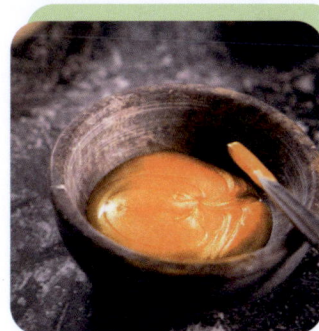

Lavender Oil & Aloe Vera Scar Fading Gel

Lavender oil promotes wound healing and reduces scars, while Aloe Vera soothes the skin and helps cell regeneration.

Ingredients:
- 1 tbsp Aloe Vera gel
- 3-4 drops lavender essential oil

Instructions:
1. Mix Aloe Vera gel with lavender oil.
2. Apply gently to scarred or healing areas.
3. Use daily for best results.

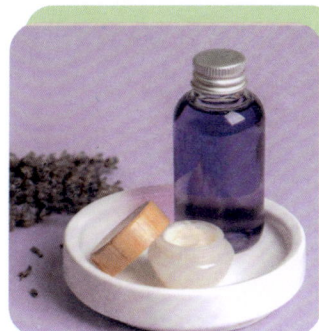

Pomegranate & Turmeric Scar Treatment

Pomegranate is rich in antioxidants that help with skin regeneration, and turmeric's curcumin supports the fading of dark marks.

Ingredients:
- 1 tbsp pomegranate seed oil
- 1/2 tsp turmeric powder

Instructions:
1. Mix pomegranate oil with turmeric powder.
2. Apply to scars and dark spots, leaving on for 15 minutes.
3. Rinse with warm water. Use 2-3 times a week.

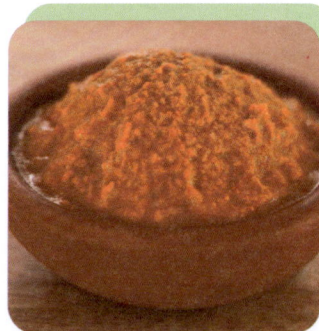

Joint & Bone Health

Support strong joints and bones – uncover the best foods and herbs to enhance mobility, strength, and skeletal health.

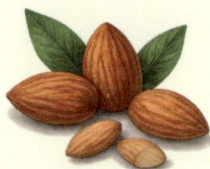

Almonds

Almonds are rich in magnesium and calcium, both essential minerals for maintaining bone strength and density. The vitamin E in almonds acts as a powerful antioxidant, reducing inflammation around the joints, alleviating stiffness, and supporting long-term joint health and mobility.

- Consume a handful (about 1 ounce) daily, or add chopped almonds to meals.

- Eating 60 g of almonds daily may reduce bone breakdown cells by 20%, supporting stronger bones.[121]

- Soak almonds overnight for easier digestion and better nutrient absorption, improved texture, and enhanced vitamins and minerals.

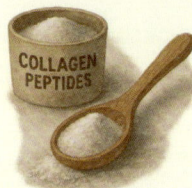

Collagen Peptides

Collagen peptides are bioavailable proteins that help rebuild cartilage and connective tissue. They also boost bone density by stimulating cells that form new bone. Collagen helps reduce stiffness, ease joint pain, and improve mobility in those with arthritis or age-related joint decline.

- Take 10 grams daily, mixed in water or smoothies for best absorption.

- Taking 5 grams of collagen peptides daily for one year increased bone mineral density in postmenopausal women.[122]

- Consume with vitamin C-rich foods (like oranges) to boost collagen synthesis, enhance skin elasticity, and support joint and bone health.

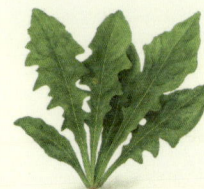

Dandelion Greens

Dandelion greens are rich in calcium and vitamin C, key nutrients for supporting bone density. Their anti-inflammatory compounds help ease joint pain and improve flexibility, while antioxidants protect bone and joint tissue from oxidative stress, damage, and inflammation.

- Add 1 cup of fresh dandelion greens to salads or smoothies daily.

- A cup of dandelion greens provides about 10% of your daily recommended calcium and over 500% of vitamin K.[123]

- Blanching the greens helps reduce bitterness while retaining nutrients for a milder taste.

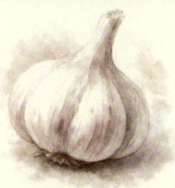

Garlic

Garlic contains sulfur compounds that reduce inflammation and protect cartilage. It may also boost estrogen levels, helping to slow bone loss and strengthen bones, especially in older adults. Its anti-inflammatory effects ease joint pain, reduce stiffness, and support overall joint health.

- Consume 1-2 raw cloves daily, or add to meals for a subtle flavor boost.

- 1,000 mg of garlic daily for 12 weeks reduced knee pain by 26% in overweight women with osteoarthritis.[124]

- Crush garlic and let it sit for 10 minutes before use to activate its beneficial sulfur compounds.

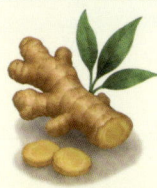

Ginger

Ginger contains gingerol, a bioactive compound that has powerful anti-inflammatory and antioxidant effects, making it effective for joint pain and swelling. Studies show ginger can inhibit compounds associated with cartilage breakdown, preserving joint health over time.

- Consume 1-2 grams of fresh ginger or ginger tea daily for maximum benefit.

- Taking 500 mg of ginger extract twice daily for six weeks reduced osteoarthritis pain by 30% vs. placebo.[125]

- Combine ginger with turmeric for a synergistic anti-inflammatory boost, especially in teas or smoothies.

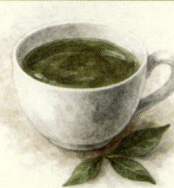

Green Tea

Green tea is rich in polyphenols, particularly EGCG, a compound that reduces joint inflammation and protects against cartilage degradation, offering relief from arthritis symptoms. Its antioxidants combat oxidative stress, helping to prevent further joint damage and support long-term joint health.

- Drink 2-3 cups of green tea daily for best results.

- 500 mg of green tea polyphenols daily for 24 weeks boosted bone formation markers by 17% in postmenopausal women.[126]

- Add a slice of lemon to boost antioxidant absorption by up to 80% and enhance detoxification, flavor, and hydration naturally.

Joint & Bone Health

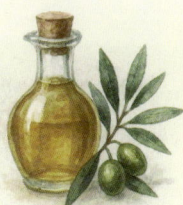

Olive Oil

Olive oil contains oleocanthal, a natural anti-inflammatory compound similar to ibuprofen in its action, which helps reduce joint pain and stiffness. Its monounsaturated fats improve bone density by enhancing calcium absorption, supporting joint flexibility, and protecting against bone loss.

- Take 1-2 tablespoons of extra virgin olive oil daily in meals or as a dressing.

- Adding extra-virgin olive oil to a Mediterranean diet for over two years raised osteocalcin levels by 51% in elderly men.[127]

- Combine with leafy greens to increase vitamin K absorption, essential for bone health.

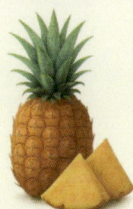

Pineapple

Pineapple is a natural source of bromelain, a powerful enzyme with anti-inflammatory properties that can help relieve arthritis-related pain and reduce swelling. Over time, bromelain also supports cartilage repair, enhances joint mobility, and promotes healthier overall joint function.

- Consume 1 cup of fresh pineapple or 100-200 mg of bromelain extract daily.

- Taking 500 mg of bromelain twice daily for six weeks cut osteoarthritis pain by 30% vs. placebo.[128]

- Eat fresh pineapple; canning reduces bromelain levels significantly and diminishes its anti-inflammatory and digestive benefits.

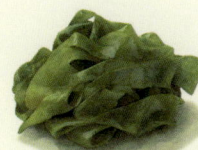

Seaweed

Seaweed is rich in minerals, and anti-inflammatory compounds like fucoidans, which help reduce joint pain, support cartilage health, and strengthen bones. It also provides essential trace minerals that aid in maintaining joint flexibility and bone density.

- Aim for 1–2 servings (5–10 g dried) of edible seaweed per week.

- One study found that daily seaweed extract eased knee osteoarthritis symptoms, with a higher dose improving symptoms by 52%.[129]

- Pairing fucoidan-rich seaweed with vitamin D enhances your body's absorption of calcium and magnesium.

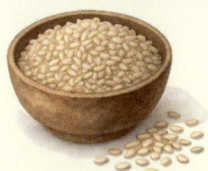

Sesame Seeds

Sesame seeds are packed with calcium, magnesium, and zinc, all essential for maintaining strong bones. Their anti-inflammatory and antioxidant properties also support joint health by reducing pain, swelling, and stiffness associated with arthritis, while promoting flexibility, mobility, and long-term bone strength.

- Consume 1-2 tablespoons of sesame seeds daily, either whole or ground.

- 40 g of sesame seeds daily for two months reduced knee pain by 63% in osteoarthritis patients.[130]

- Soak seeds overnight to enhance nutrient absorption, particularly calcium, and improve digestion, texture, and overall bioavailability.

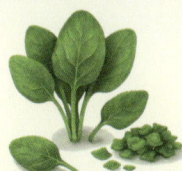

Spinach

Spinach is high in vitamin K, calcium, and magnesium, all essential for maintaining bone strength and density. Its antioxidants, such as lutein, help reduce joint pain and stiffness. Regular consumption of spinach may also help slow age-related bone loss and support overall joint health.

- Eat 1-2 cups of spinach daily, either raw in salads or lightly cooked.

- Regular spinach intake is associated with a 10% increase in bone mineral density.[131]

- Cook lightly to increase the bioavailability of calcium and magnesium, and enhance nutrient absorption.

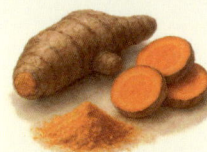

Turmeric

Turmeric's active compound, curcumin, has powerful anti-inflammatory effects that help reduce joint swelling, stiffness, and alleviate pain associated with arthritis. It works by blocking inflammatory cytokines and enzymes that contribute to arthritis symptoms, joint damage, and decreased mobility.

- Take 500-1000 mg of curcumin or 1/2 teaspoon of turmeric daily.

- Taking 1,000 mg of curcumin daily for 8–12 weeks reduced osteoarthritis pain, comparable to NSAIDs.[132]

- Pair with black pepper; it enhances curcumin absorption by up to 2000% and boosts turmeric's anti-inflammatory and antioxidant effects.

Arthritis Relief

EXTRA HERBS

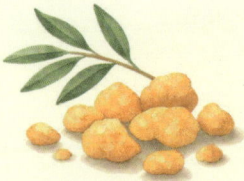

Boswellia

Boswellia contains anti-inflammatory compounds, especially boswellic acids, that help reduce pain and improve joint function in arthritis by inhibiting pro-inflammatory enzymes.

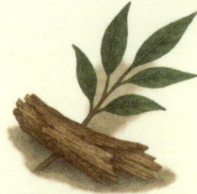

Willow Bark

Willow bark, known as "nature's aspirin," contains salicin, a natural compound that helps reduce inflammation and relieve pain associated with arthritis, joint stiffness, and muscle soreness.

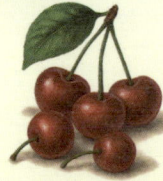

Cherries (Tart Cherry Extract)

Tart cherry extract is rich in anthocyanins with strong anti-inflammatory effects. It may help reduce joint pain, stiffness, and swelling, particularly in gout-related arthritis.

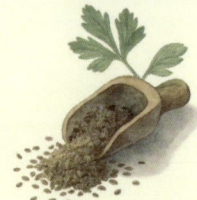

Celery Seeds

Celery seeds contain antioxidants and anti-inflammatory compounds like luteolin. They support joint health by reducing inflammation and easing arthritis-related pain.

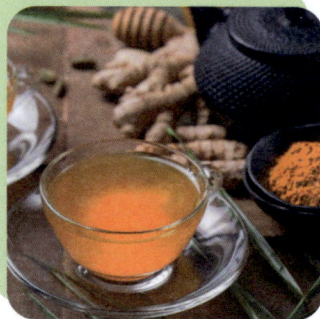

Golden Anti-Inflammatory Tea

This tea blends anti-inflammatory turmeric and ginger with olive oil for better absorption. It's a warming, soothing drink that may help ease joint pain and stiffness.

Ingredients:
- 1 cup water
- 1/2 tsp turmeric powder
- 1/2 tsp freshly grated ginger
- 1 tsp olive oil
- 1 tsp honey (optional, for taste)

Instructions:
1. Boil water and add turmeric and ginger. Let it simmer for 5 minutes.
2. Remove from heat and add olive oil and honey (if desired). Stir well.
3. Drink warm once daily to support joint health.

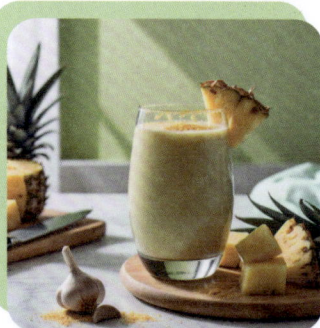

Garlic & Pineapple Smoothie

Garlic has been shown to reduce inflammatory markers, and pineapple contains bromelain, an enzyme known for its anti-inflammatory and pain-relieving properties. This refreshing smoothie is a tasty way to relieve arthritis symptoms.

Ingredients:
- 1 cup fresh pineapple chunks
- 1 clove garlic, minced
- 1/2 cup almond milk
- 1/4 tsp turmeric powder (optional for extra anti-inflammatory boost)

Instructions:
1. Add pineapple, garlic, almond milk, and turmeric (if using) to a blender.
2. Blend until smooth.
3. Enjoy this smoothie in the morning to help manage arthritis pain.

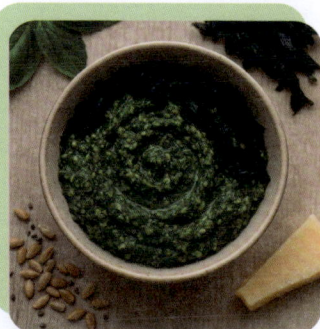

Seaweed Pesto

This seaweed pesto is rich in iodine for thyroid support, plus minerals and prebiotic fiber for gut health. Blended with herbs, nuts, and olive oil, it's a nourishing and flavorful addition to any meal.

Ingredients:
- 1 cup fresh basil or parsley
- 2 tbsp seaweed flakes (or ¼ cup soaked whole pieces)
- ¼ cup sunflower seeds, cashews, or pine nuts
- 1–2 garlic cloves
- ¼ cup Parmesan or nutritional yeast (optional)
- 2–3 tbsp lemon juice
- ⅓ cup olive oil (more as needed)
- Salt & pepper to taste

Instructions:
1. Soak whole seaweed 5–10 mins if using; drain and squeeze dry.
2. Add basil, seaweed, nuts, garlic, cheese/yeast, and lemon juice to a food processor.
3. Pulse, then blend while slowly adding olive oil until desired consistency.
4. Season with salt and pepper, and blend again.
5. Store in a sealed jar in the fridge for up to 5 days, or freeze in portions.

Bone Density & Osteoporosis

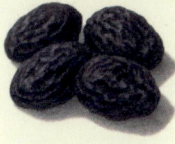

Prunes

Prunes are rich in boron and potassium, minerals essential for bone health. Studies show they may help reduce the risk of osteoporosis, and support long-term skeletal strength and density.

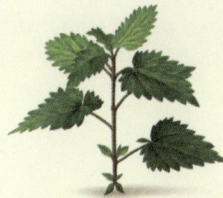

Nettle Leaf

Nettle leaf provides calcium, magnesium, and other bone-supportive minerals. Research suggests it may help maintain or improve bone density, especially in postmenopausal women.

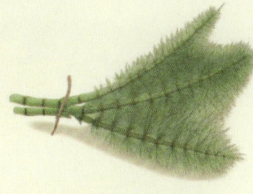

Horsetail

Horsetail is high in silica, a key mineral for bone growth and density. It supports calcium absorption and helps strengthen bones, connective tissue, and overall skeletal structure.

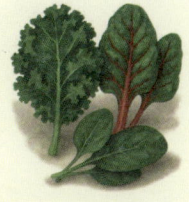

Vitamin K-Rich Greens

Greens like kale and spinach are rich in vitamin K, which is vital for producing osteocalcin—a protein that binds calcium to bones, improving density and structural strength.

Almond & Sesame Bone-Boosting Milk

Almonds and sesame seeds are high in calcium and magnesium, essential minerals for bone density. This delicious homemade milk provides a bone-strengthening nutrient boost, ideal for osteoporosis support.

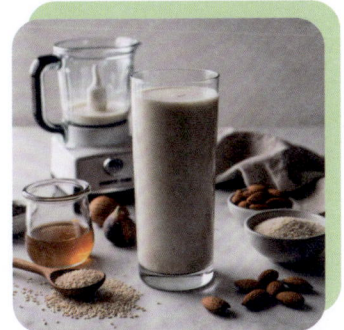

Ingredients:

- 1/4 cup almonds, soaked overnight
- 1 tbsp sesame seeds, soaked overnight
- 1 cup water
- 1 tsp honey (optional, for taste)

Instructions:

1. Drain and rinse almonds and sesame seeds.
2. Blend with water until smooth, then strain if desired.
3. Add honey for sweetness, and drink this daily to support bone density.

Dandelion & Spinach Mineral Salad

Dandelion greens and spinach are rich in calcium and vitamin K, which are crucial for bone strength. This mineral-packed salad helps replenish bone-supportive nutrients, especially when paired with olive oil for nutrient absorption.

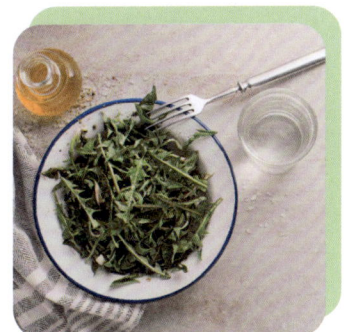

Ingredients:

- 1 cup fresh dandelion greens
- 1/2 cup spinach leaves
- 1 tbsp olive oil
- 1 tbsp lemon juice
- Salt and pepper to taste

Instructions:

1. Toss dandelion greens and spinach with olive oil, lemon juice, salt, and pepper.
2. Enjoy this salad daily as a mineral boost for stronger bones.

Pineapple & Green Tea Bone-Strength Smoothie

This refreshing smoothie pairs pineapple, known for its enzymes that may aid in calcium absorption, with green tea, which is rich in antioxidants that promote bone health. It's a delicious way to maintain bone density and strength.

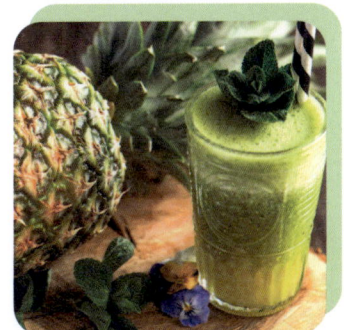

Ingredients:

- 1 cup fresh pineapple chunks
- 1/2 cup brewed green tea, cooled
- 1/4 cup almond milk
- 1 tsp honey (optional)

Instructions:

1. Add all ingredients to a blender and blend until smooth.
2. Enjoy this smoothie in the morning or as a snack for a bone-strengthening boost.

Pain Relief

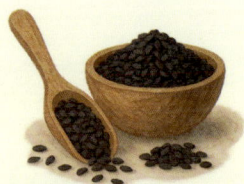

Black Cumin (Nigella sativa)

Black cumin contains strong natural compounds, especially thymoquinone, that help lower inflammation and ease pain. It can reduce joint pain, swelling, and stiffness by calming the body's response to inflammation and blocking pain signals.

- Massage a few drops of black cumin oil directly onto sore joints 2–3 times per week.

- Black cumin oil cut knee pain by 34% and improved function by 28%, far outperforming placebo in osteoarthritis patients.[133]

- Choose cold-pressed black cumin seed oil for the highest potency, and store it in a cool, dark place to preserve its anti-inflammatory properties.

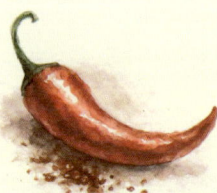

Cayenne Pepper

Cayenne contains capsaicin, which works by blocking pain signals to the brain and reducing inflammation in affected areas. This action can be particularly effective for nerve pain and chronic conditions like arthritis by desensitizing pain receptors over time.

- Add a pinch to meals or mix 1/4 teaspoon with a carrier oil to apply topically on sore areas.

- Topical capsaicin reduced osteoarthritis pain by about 50% after four weeks of use.[134]

- Start with a low dose and increase gradually to build tolerance; combining with ginger enhances anti-inflammatory effects.

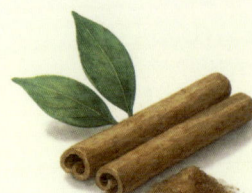

Cinnamon

Cinnamon is rich in cinnamaldehyde and proanthocyanidins, which have anti-inflammatory and antioxidant effects that target pain and stiffness, particularly in joints. It also promotes blood circulation, which aids muscle recovery and reduces pain over time.

- Mix 1/2 teaspoon of cinnamon powder into warm water with honey, consume once daily.

- Cinnamon was found to reduce pain and shorten its duration in people with menstrual cramps.[135]

- Use Ceylon cinnamon for maximum benefit, as it has stronger anti-inflammatory properties and is gentler on the liver.

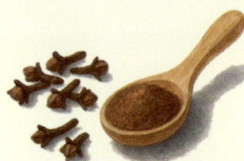

Cloves

Cloves contain eugenol, a powerful natural anesthetic with strong anti-inflammatory properties that help numb pain and reduce swelling. Its analgesic effects make it especially effective for relieving toothaches, soothing muscle pain, easing minor discomforts, and supporting oral health.

- For toothaches, place a clove on the affected area; for muscle pain, massage diluted clove oil onto sore muscles.

- Clove gel can provide pain relief comparable to benzocaine during dental needle insertions.[136]

- Use whole cloves for toothaches as they release eugenol slowly; for muscle pain, warm the oil slightly for better absorption.

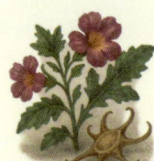

Devil's Claw

Devil's Claw contains harpagoside, a potent anti-inflammatory compound that helps reduce joint pain, stiffness, and swelling, particularly in conditions like osteoarthritis and chronic back pain. It may also improve mobility, joint function, flexibility, endurance, and overall physical comfort and quality of life.

- Simmer 1–2 teaspoons dried Devil's Claw root for 10–15 minutes; drink 1 cup once or twice daily.

- A study found 12 weeks of Devil's Claw extract reduced pain by 23.8% and stiffness by 22.2% in hip or knee osteoarthritis.[137]

- Always simmer the root (don't just steep) to extract the active compounds, enhance potency, and ensure maximum benefits.

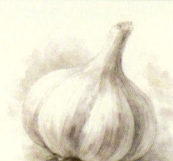

Garlic

Garlic's sulfur compounds, such as allicin, offer potent anti-inflammatory effects that help relieve joint and muscle pain. It also enhances blood flow, supports healing in inflamed areas, reduces oxidative stress, and eases chronic pain over time, improving mobility, flexibility, and overall physical well-being.

- Consume 1-2 raw cloves daily or add minced garlic to meals.

- 400 mg of garlic extract daily can alleviate endometriosis-related pain within three months.[138]

- Crush garlic and let it sit for 10 minutes to maximize allicin production, boost its healing power, and enhance anti-inflammatory benefits.

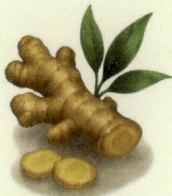

Pain Relief

Ginger

Ginger contains gingerol and zingerone, compounds known for their anti-inflammatory and pain-relieving properties. It is effective in reducing muscle soreness, joint pain, and the frequency of migraine attacks, as it inhibits key pain pathways in the body.

- Brew a 1-inch piece of fresh ginger for tea or take 1/2 teaspoon powdered ginger daily.

- 500 mg of ginger powder three times daily for the first three days of menstruation can ease pain significantly.[139]

- For faster migraine relief, chew on a fresh ginger slice; combine with turmeric to enhance anti-inflammatory effects.

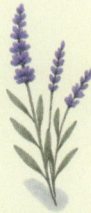

Lavender

Lavender contains linalool and linalyl acetate, which soothe the nervous system, easing muscle tension and headaches. Its anti-inflammatory effects reduce pain, while inhaling it calms the mind, lowers stress, and promotes relaxation that can lessen overall discomfort.

- Use 2-3 drops of lavender oil in a diffuser, or add a few fresh lavender sprigs to hot water for inhalation.

- Inhaling 1% lavender oil can significantly reduce sensory pain in postherpetic neuralgia patients by 7.07 points.[140]

- Rub diluted lavender oil on temples to soothe headache pain quickly, reduce tension, promote relaxation, and calm the nervous system.

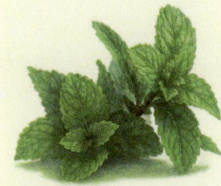

Peppermint

Peppermint contains menthol, which relaxes muscles and provides a cooling sensation, ideal for relieving tension headaches and muscle soreness. It also acts as a natural analgesic by desensitizing pain receptors, providing relief from nerve pain, inflammation, and discomfort.

- Apply diluted peppermint oil to temples and neck, or steep fresh leaves in hot water for tea.

- Inhaling peppermint essential oil post-surgery can reduce pain severity by 29%.[141]

- For migraines, apply peppermint oil under the nostrils for fast relief, reduced sensitivity to light, eased tension, and improved airflow.

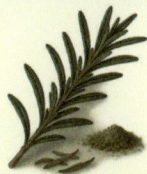

Rosemary

Rosemary contains carnosic and rosmarinic acids, which reduce inflammation and boost circulation, easing muscle pain and cramps. Its warming effect stimulates blood flow, aiding recovery and reducing stiffness, while antioxidants support cellular healing, tissue repair, muscle relaxation, and overall muscle health and resilience.

- Apply rosemary-infused oil on sore muscles or use dried rosemary leaves to make tea.

- Massaging with rosemary oil twice daily can reduce chronic shoulder pain by 30%.[142]

- Add rosemary to a warm bath to enhance its muscle-relieving effects, boost circulation, ease tension, and promote deep relaxation.

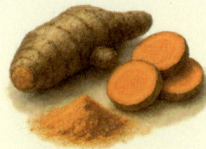

Turmeric

Turmeric's active compound, curcumin, inhibits inflammation pathways, making it highly effective for joint and muscle pain. Curcumin also aids in tissue repair, supports recovery from injuries and chronic pain conditions, and promotes overall healing. Black pepper boosts its absorption by 2000%.

- Take 1 teaspoon of turmeric with a pinch of black pepper in warm milk or water daily.

- Taking 500 mg of turmeric extract twice daily can relieve knee osteoarthritis pain as effectively as paracetamol.[143]

- For faster relief, mix turmeric with coconut oil and apply it as a paste to the affected area.

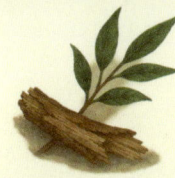

Willow Bark

Willow bark contains salicin, a compound similar to aspirin, that reduces pain and inflammation. It is particularly effective for back pain, arthritis, and headaches. Its anti-inflammatory effects provide prolonged relief, as it metabolizes slowly in the body, promoting steady, natural pain management.

- Drink willow bark tea or take 1-2 capsules of powdered bark daily.

- Taking willow bark extract with 240 mg salicin daily can reduce osteoarthritis pain by 14% in two weeks.[144]

- Avoid combining with other NSAIDs, as it enhances their effects, potentially leading to overstimulation.

Muscle & Chronic Pain Relief

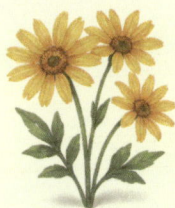

Arnica

Arnica is widely used for its anti-inflammatory and pain-relieving properties. It helps reduce muscle soreness, bruising, and swelling, and is commonly applied topically in creams or gels.

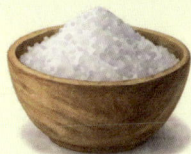

Epsom Salt

Epsom salt is rich in magnesium, which helps ease muscle tension, reduce inflammation, and relieve soreness. Adding it to warm baths can be beneficial for chronic pain relief.

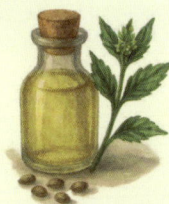

Hemp Seed Oil

Hemp seed oil contains essential fatty acids and anti-inflammatory compounds that reduce muscle stiffness and pain. It can be used topically or taken internally for ongoing support.

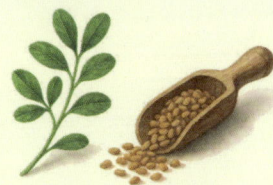

Fenugreek

Fenugreek has natural anti-inflammatory effects that can help relieve pain and swelling. It's traditionally used as a tea or supplement to ease muscle discomfort and chronic conditions.

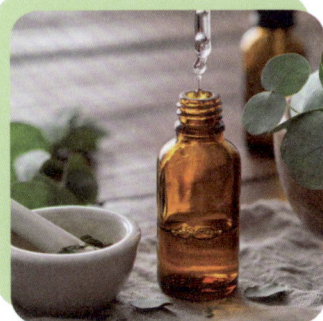

Peppermint & Eucalyptus Muscle Rub

Peppermint and eucalyptus oils contain natural menthol and eucalyptol, which create a cooling sensation that soothes sore muscles and alleviates stiffness. This blend is ideal for massage after physical exertion.

Ingredients:
- 5 drops peppermint essential oil
- 5 drops eucalyptus essential oil
- 2 tbsp coconut oil

Instructions:
1. Mix the oils in a small bowl until well combined.
2. Massage the blend onto sore muscles in circular motions.
3. Leave it on for at least 30 minutes, then rinse if desired.

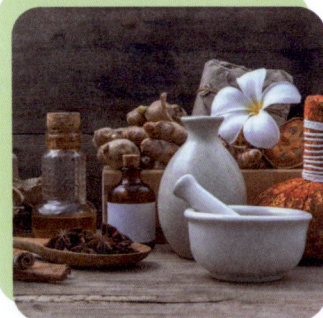

Cinnamon & Clove Warm Compress

Cinnamon and clove are known for their warming and analgesic properties. Together, they promote circulation and relieve deep muscle pain when applied directly with heat.

Ingredients:
- 1 tsp cinnamon powder
- 1 tsp ground cloves
- 1 cup warm water
- Small cloth or compress

Instructions:
1. Mix cinnamon and cloves with warm water in a small bowl.
2. Soak a cloth in the mixture, wring out excess water, and apply it to the sore area.
3. Leave the compress on for 10-15 minutes, repeating as needed for relief.

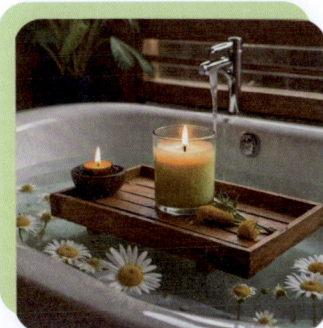

Arnica & Epsom Salt Soothing Bath Soak

Arnica has natural anti-inflammatory and analgesic properties that, when combined with magnesium-rich Epsom salts, work to relax muscles and relieve pain. This bath soak is ideal for easing chronic muscle pain after a long day.

Ingredients:
- 1 cup Epsom salt
- 1 tbsp arnica gel or 1 tbsp dried arnica flowers
- 10 drops lavender essential oil (optional)
- Warm water in a bathtub

Instructions:
1. Fill the bathtub with warm water and add the Epsom salt and arnica.
2. Stir in lavender oil for added relaxation benefits.
3. Soak in the bath for 20-30 minutes, allowing the ingredients to ease muscle soreness.
4. Rinse off and pat dry.

Headaches, Migraines, & Nerve Pain

EXTRA HERBS

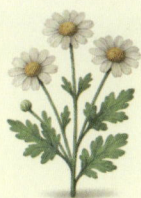

Feverfew

Feverfew is a well-researched herb used for migraine and headache relief. It contains compounds that reduce inflammation, help block pain signals in the brain, and may prevent migraine episodes.

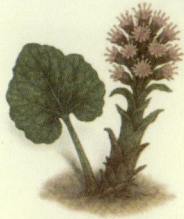

Butterbur

Butterbur contains petasin and isopetasin, which help reduce the frequency and severity of migraines. It's commonly taken as a supplement for long-term headache relief, and reduced inflammation in the brain.

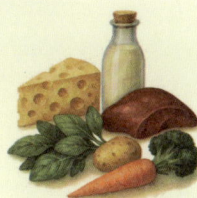

Riboflavin

Riboflavin (vitamin B2) has been shown to lower migraine frequency by improving mitochondrial function. It's found in foods like almonds, eggs, and leafy green vegetables.

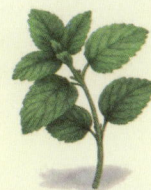

Lemon Balm

Lemon balm has calming and anti-inflammatory effects that can ease stress-related headaches and nerve pain. It can be consumed as tea or taken as a supplement daily or as needed.

Lavender & Basil Inhalation

Lavender and basil are renowned for their calming and analgesic properties, making this inhalation method effective for easing headaches and calming nerves.

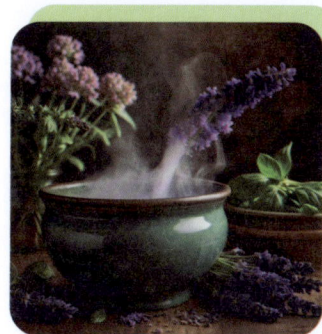

Ingredients:
- 5 drops lavender essential oil
- 2 fresh basil leaves (or 2 drops basil essential oil)
- Hot water in a bowl

Instructions:
1. Add the lavender and basil to a bowl of hot water.
2. Lean over the bowl with a towel over your head to trap the steam.
3. Inhale deeply for 5-10 minutes to relax muscles and relieve tension.

Peppermint & Willow Bark Headache Balm

Peppermint and willow bark are ideal for headache relief. The menthol in peppermint oil provides a cooling sensation, while willow bark's salicin content works as a natural pain reliever.

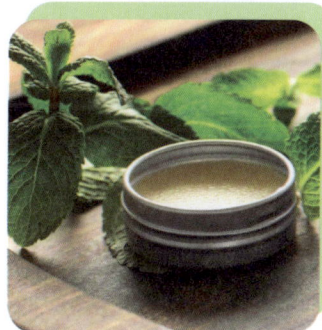

Ingredients:
- 5 drops peppermint essential oil
- 1 tsp willow bark powder (available in health stores or online)
- 1 tbsp olive oil

Instructions:
1. Mix peppermint oil, willow bark powder, and olive oil in a small bowl.
2. Massage a small amount onto temples and the back of the neck.
3. Leave it on as the balm cools and soothes.

Lemon Balm & Feverfew Headache-Relief Tea

Lemon balm and feverfew have been used traditionally for their calming and pain-relieving effects, particularly for headaches and migraines. Lemon balm helps to reduce stress and tension, while feverfew is known for its ability to alleviate migraine symptoms.

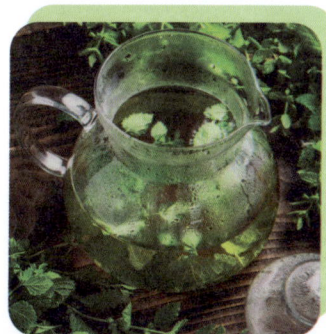

Ingredients:
- 1 tsp dried lemon balm leaves
- 1 tsp dried feverfew leaves
- 1 cup boiling water
- 1 tsp honey (optional)

Instructions:
1. Place the lemon balm and feverfew in a tea infuser or directly in a cup.
2. Pour boiling water over the herbs and let steep for 10 minutes.
3. Remove the herbs, add honey if desired, and sip slowly.
4. Enjoy as needed to relieve headache symptoms.

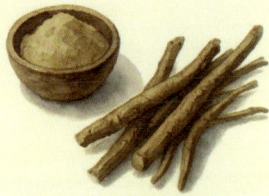

Women's Health

Ashwagandha

Ashwagandha is an adaptogen known for its ability to reduce cortisol, helping to balance hormones and ease menopausal symptoms. It has been shown to enhance reproductive health by supporting ovarian function, improving fertility markers, and boosting overall vitality naturally.

Take 300-500 mg of ashwagandha extract daily, or 1-2 teaspoon of powder in warm milk or tea.

300 mg of ashwagandha root extract twice daily for eight weeks improved women's sexual function scores by 57%.[145]

Use consistently for best results; pair with turmeric for enhanced stress relief, hormonal support, and improved overall well-being.

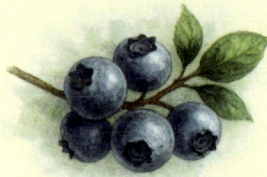

Blueberries

Blueberries are packed with flavonoids, which help maintain balanced estrogen levels and protect cells from oxidative stress. Their high antioxidant content supports heart health and skin elasticity, particularly beneficial during menopause.

Consume 1/2 to 1 cup of fresh or frozen blueberries daily.

150 g of blueberries daily for six months improved blood vessel function by 1.1% and cut systolic pressure by 5 mmHg.[146]

Pair with a source of healthy fat, like almonds, to boost absorption of fat-soluble vitamins, support hormone production, and enhance nutrients.

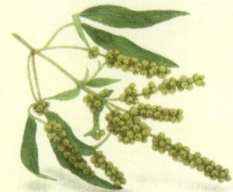

Chasteberry

Chasteberry balances prolactin, easing menstrual issues and supporting fertility. It boosts progesterone, reducing PMS symptoms like bloating, tenderness, and mood swings. It's especially helpful for irregular cycles, menopause transition, and hormonal imbalance recovery.

Take 400 mg of Vitex extract or 20-40 mg of dried fruit daily.

Taking 20 mg of chasteberry daily for three months reduced PMS symptoms, with 93% of women reporting improvement.[147]

Works best when taken in the morning; avoid pairing with hormonal medications for optimal effect, and balanced absorption.

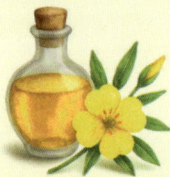

Evening Primrose Oil

Evening primrose oil is rich in gamma-linolenic acid (GLA), which can reduce hot flashes, breast pain, and mood disturbances associated with menopause. It also supports skin health by improving moisture levels, reducing acne linked to hormonal imbalances, and promoting overall hormonal stability.

Take 500-1,000 mg of evening primrose oil daily, ideally with meals.

500 mg of evening primrose oil twice daily for six weeks reduced hot flash severity by 42% in menopausal women.[148]

For skin benefits, try mixing a few drops into your moisturizer; keep refrigerated for freshness, potency, and extended shelf life.

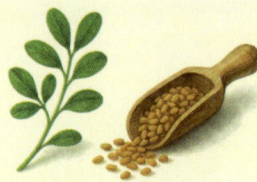

Fenugreek

Fenugreek seeds contain phytoestrogens that support healthy estrogen levels, enhancing libido and promoting menstrual health. They help boost breast milk production, ease cramps and bloating, regulate blood sugar, support metabolic function, and aid hormone balance in women with irregular cycles.

Take 500-1,000 mg of fenugreek supplement or 1-2 teaspoons of seeds daily in warm water.

250 mg of fenugreek twice daily for 42 days boosted sexual function by 41.6% and reduced irritability by 40%.[149]

Steep seeds overnight and drink the water for a gentle, effective daily dose that supports digestion, hormonal balance, and overall wellness.

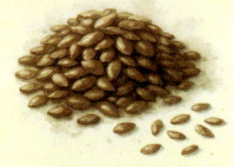

Flaxseed

Flaxseeds are high in lignans, which mimic estrogen and help balance hormones. They help alleviate hot flashes and mood swings during menopause and support regular menstrual cycles. The omega-3s in flaxseeds also promote hormonal health, reduce inflammation, and support overall well-being.

Consume 1-2 tablespoons of ground flaxseed daily.

Consuming 40 g of flaxseed daily for three months cut total cholesterol by 9% and LDL by 12% in postmenopausal women.[150]

Grind flaxseeds fresh for maximum nutrient absorption; store in the fridge to prevent oxidation, preserve freshness.

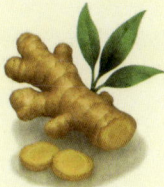

Women's Health

Ginger

Ginger is a natural anti-inflammatory that alleviates menstrual cramps by reducing prostaglandins, compounds responsible for pain and inflammation. It also aids in digestion, reducing bloating and nausea during menstrual cycles, and supports hormonal balance.

Drink ginger tea (1–2 teaspoons grated ginger in hot water) or take 500 mg ginger powder.

1,500 mg of ginger powder daily for three days during menstruation offers pain relief comparable to NSAIDs.[151]

Pair with honey for an extra soothing effect; fresh ginger works better than dried for pain relief.

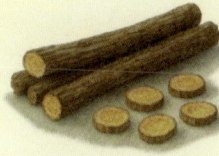

Licorice Root

Licorice root contains phytoestrogens that help balance estrogen and progesterone, alleviating symptoms of menopause such as hot flashes and mood swings. It also supports adrenal health, helping to reduce stress, balance cortisol levels, and promote hormonal harmony.

Drink 1 cup of licorice root tea daily or take 250 mg of licorice root extract.

1.5 g of licorice extract daily with a low-calorie diet for 8 weeks reduced weight and waist size in women with PCOS.[152]

Avoid prolonged use; take breaks after 2-3 weeks to prevent any effects on blood pressure.

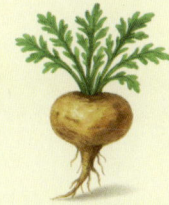

Maca Root

Maca root, an adaptogen, helps regulate hormones by supporting the endocrine system. It's widely used to improve libido, fertility, and energy levels, especially during menopause when estrogen levels dip. Maca also enhances mood, reduces anxiety, and promotes overall hormonal balance.

Start with 1 teaspoon of maca powder daily, and gradually increase to 1 tablespoon.

Taking 3.3 g daily for 12 weeks significantly lowered diastolic blood pressure in postmenopausal women.[153]

Use gelatinized maca for easier digestion and absorption, especially for sensitive stomachs.

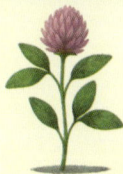

Red Clover

Red clover contains isoflavones, compounds that mimic estrogen, helping to reduce hot flashes and night sweats during menopause. It also supports bone density, cardiovascular health, and hormonal balance, making it especially beneficial for women as they age and experience declining hormone levels.

Take 40 mg of red clover extract daily or drink a cup of red clover tea.

Red clover isoflavone supplements can reduce hot flashes by about 1.73 episodes daily in postmenopausal women.[154]

Try red clover tea in the evening to promote restful sleep, ease nighttime symptoms, and support hormonal balance while you rest.

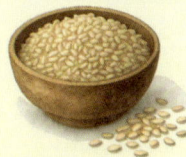

Sesame Seeds

Sesame seeds are rich in lignans, natural plant compounds that act like phytoestrogens, helping to balance hormones, especially during menopause. They also support bone health with calcium and magnesium, and improve cholesterol levels, antioxidant status, and overall hormonal well-being.

Aim for 1–2 tablespoons (10–20 g) of sesame seeds per day.

50 g of sesame seeds daily for 5 weeks increased hormone-binding protein by 15% and a hormone marker by 72%.[155]

Grind whole sesame seeds in a spice grinder or mortar and pestle before eating to unlock their nutrients, and enhance their health benefits.

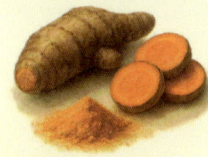

Turmeric

Turmeric's active compound, curcumin, the active ingredient in turmeric, reduces inflammation and is especially helpful for relieving menstrual pain and regulating cycles. It also aids in detoxifying the liver, which is crucial for healthy hormone metabolism and overall reproductive system balance.

Add 1/2 teaspoon of turmeric powder to warm milk with a pinch of black pepper daily.

Taking 100 mg of curcumin twice daily for 10 days each cycle reduced PMS symptoms.[156]

Use turmeric root paste in cooking for a richer flavor, enhanced absorption, and a powerful health boost.

Menopause & Hormonal Balance

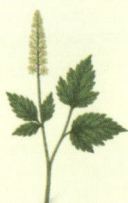

Black Cohosh

Black cohosh contains triterpene glycosides that help reduce hot flashes, night sweats, and mood swings. It supports hormonal balance by interacting with serotonin receptors.

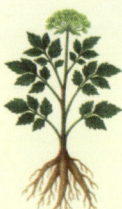

Dong Quai

Dong quai, often called "female ginseng," contains phytoestrogens that help balance estrogen levels. It may reduce hot flashes and support hormonal stability during menopause.

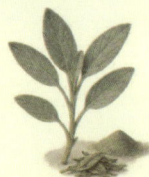

Sage

Sage is rich in rosmarinic acid and antioxidants. It helps reduce hot flashes and supports cognitive function, both commonly affected during menopause and hormonal changes.

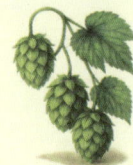

Hops

Hops contain phytoestrogens like 8-prenylnaringenin, which mimic estrogen activity. They help ease menopausal symptoms such as hot flashes, promote better sleep, and support hormonal balance.

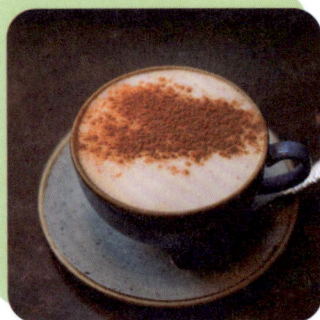

Hormone Harmony Latte

Ashwagandha and maca root are powerful adaptogens that support stress management and hormonal balance. Fenugreek adds phytoestrogens to aid in alleviating menopause symptoms, while the almond milk base provides a creamy and nourishing touch.

Ingredients:
- 1 cup unsweetened almond milk
- 1 tsp ashwagandha powder
- 1 tsp maca root powder
- 1/2 tsp fenugreek powder
- Honey or maple syrup to taste (optional)

Instructions:
1. Heat almond milk in a saucepan until warm, not boiling.
2. Add ashwagandha, maca root, and fenugreek powders, stirring well to combine.
3. Sweeten with honey or maple syrup if desired.
4. Pour into a mug and enjoy this calming, hormone-balancing latte.

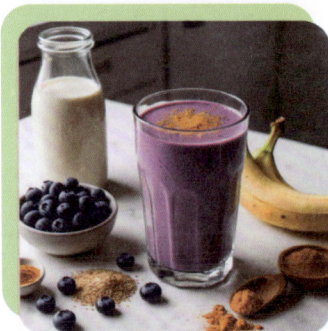

Menopause Relief Smoothie

This smoothie combines hormone-supportive ingredients like flaxseed and blueberries, which are rich in antioxidants and phytoestrogens that can help reduce hot flashes and support overall hormonal health.

Ingredients:
- 1 cup almond milk
- 1/2 cup blueberries (fresh or frozen)
- 1 tbsp ground flaxseed
- 1 tsp turmeric powder
- 1/2 banana for creaminess

Instructions:
1. Combine all ingredients in a blender and blend until smooth.
2. Pour into a glass and enjoy as a refreshing and hormone-supportive drink.

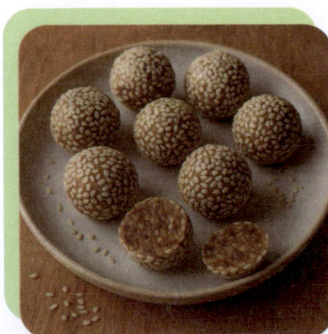

Sesame Seed & Date Hormone-Balancing Bites

Sesame seeds offer calcium, magnesium, and lignans that support hormones, bones, and PMS relief. Paired with dates and almond butter, these bites deliver lasting energy and key nutrients for women's wellness.

Ingredients (Makes ~10 bites):
- ½ cup pitted Medjool dates
- ¼ cup tahini or 2 tbsp sesame + 2 tbsp almond butter
- 2 tbsp ground flaxseed (optional)
- 2 tbsp sesame seeds (plus more for coating)
- ¼ tsp cinnamon
- Pinch of sea salt
- 1 tsp honey (optional)

Instructions:
1. Blend dates in a food processor until broken down.
2. Add remaining ingredients and blend into a
3. sticky dough.
   Roll into balls, then coat in sesame seeds.
4. Chill for 30 minutes to firm.
5. Store in the fridge for up to 1 week.

Menstrual Health & Fertility

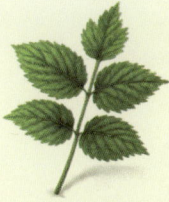

Raspberry Leaf

Raspberry leaf contains fragarine, a compound that tones and strengthens the uterine muscles. It helps reduce menstrual cramps and supports overall reproductive health.

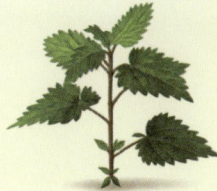

Nettle

Nettle is rich in iron and essential minerals, helping to replenish nutrients lost during menstruation. It supports energy levels, reduces fatigue, and promotes healthy, regular menstrual cycles.

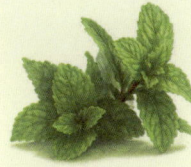

Peppermint

Peppermint contains menthol, which has natural muscle-relaxing properties. It helps ease menstrual cramps, reduce bloating, and promote digestive comfort during the menstrual cycle.

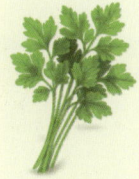

Parsley

Parsley is high in vitamin C and iron, both important for menstruation. It supports hormone synthesis, improves iron levels, reduces fatigue, and helps regulate menstrual cycles naturally.

Cinnamon & Ashwagandha PCOS-Friendly Oat Bars

These bars combine cinnamon to support blood sugar, ashwagandha to reduce stress and balance hormones, and oats, seeds, and nut butter for lasting energy and satiety—ideal for managing PCOS symptoms.

Ingredients (Makes 8–10 bars):

- 1½ cups rolled oats
- ½ cup almond or peanut butter
- ¼ cup ground flaxseed or chia seeds
- ¼ cup chopped nuts/seeds (optional)
- 2 tbsp honey or stevia (to taste)
- ½ tsp cinnamon
- ½ tsp ashwagandha powder
- 2–4 tbsp almond milk (as needed)

Instructions:

1. Mix oats, flaxseed, nuts, cinnamon, and ashwagandha in a bowl.
2. In another bowl, whisk nut butter, sweetener, and 2 tbsp almond milk.
3. Combine wet and dry; add more milk if needed for a sticky dough.
4. Press into a lined pan and chill for 1 hour.
5. Slice into bars and store in the fridge (up to 1 week) or freeze.

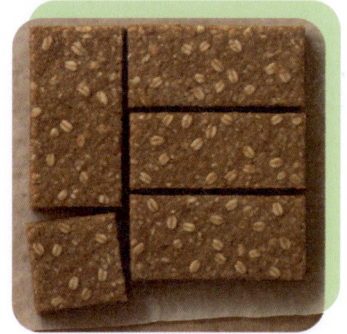

Raspberry Leaf & Nettle Fertility Tea

Raspberry leaf is renowned for toning the uterus and supporting menstrual health, while nettle provides essential vitamins and minerals that benefit reproductive health.

Ingredients:

- 1 tsp dried raspberry leaf
- 1 tsp dried nettle leaf
- 1 cup hot water
- 1 tsp honey or lemon to taste (optional)

Instructions:

1. Combine raspberry leaf and nettle in a teapot and pour hot water over them.
2. Steep for 10-15 minutes, then strain.
3. Sweeten with honey or add a splash of lemon, if desired, and enjoy this nourishing tea for menstrual support.

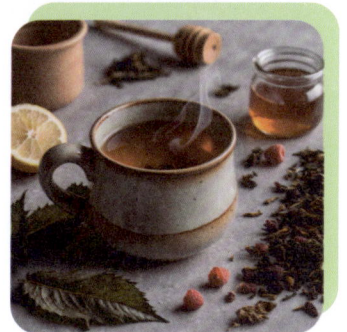

Sesame & Turmeric Crusted Salmon

This recipe pairs omega-3-rich salmon with anti-inflammatory turmeric and mineral-packed sesame seeds to support hormones, reduce PMS symptoms, and boost overall vitality.

Ingredients:

- 2 salmon fillets (5–6 oz each)
- 1 tbsp sesame seeds
- ½ tsp turmeric
- ¼ tsp black pepper
- ½ tsp garlic powder
- 1 tsp olive or sesame oil
- Sea salt to taste
- Optional: lemon wedges & parsley (garnish)

Instructions:

1. Preheat oven to 200°C (400°F) and line a tray.
2. Mix sesame seeds, spices, and salt.
3. Pat salmon dry, rub with oil, and press on spice mix.
4. Bake 12–15 mins until cooked through.
5. Serve with greens, quinoa, or sweet potato. Garnish if desired.

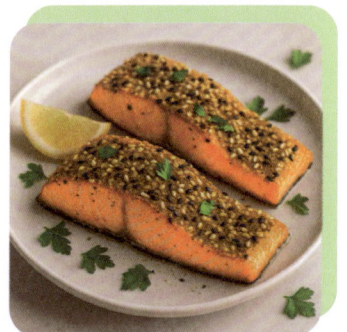

Oral Health

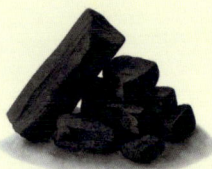

Activated Charcoal

Activated charcoal's porous structure binds to plaque, bacteria, and stain-causing compounds, helping to whiten teeth and freshen breath. It's particularly effective at absorbing tannins from coffee, tea, and wine, which can cause discoloration and dull enamel appearance.

- Use ½ teaspoon activated charcoal on a wet toothbrush; brush gently for 1–2 minutes, 1–2 times weekly.

- Using activated charcoal toothpaste can remove 28.82% more stains than regular toothpaste.[157]

- Rinse thoroughly after use to avoid charcoal residue, and avoid overuse to prevent enamel wear.

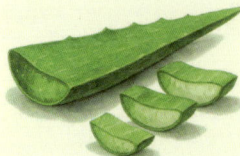

Aloe Vera

Aloe vera's natural antibacterial and anti-inflammatory properties help soothe gum inflammation and support healing. Its gentle gel reduces irritation, provides a protective barrier on sensitive tissues, and promotes healthier gums when used regularly in oral care.

- Apply pure aloe vera gel to gums and massage. Leave for 5-10 minutes before rinsing, once daily.

- Aloe vera mouthwash can reduce plaque by 35% and gingivitis by 33% in four weeks.[158]

- Use fresh aloe vera gel directly from the plant for maximum potency, soothing power, and skin-healing benefits.

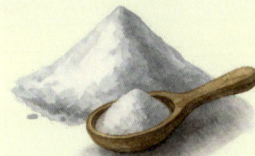

Baking Soda

Baking soda is mildly abrasive, helping to remove surface stains on teeth and break down plaque. It neutralizes acids in the mouth, balancing pH levels and preventing enamel erosion, and can reduce bad breath by minimizing odor-causing bacteria.

- Mix 1/2 teaspoon with water to create a paste. Brush teeth with the paste 2-3 times per week.

- Baking soda toothpastes can reduce plaque by 49% and gingivitis by 60% vs. non-baking soda types.[159]

- Avoid brushing too hard, it can be abrasive. For an extra fresh kick, add a drop of peppermint oil.

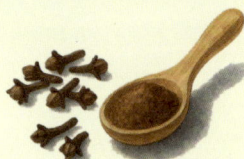

Clove

Clove contains eugenol, a natural anesthetic and antiseptic that helps reduce tooth pain and kill harmful bacteria in the mouth. Its anti-inflammatory properties make it effective for gum health, relieving swelling, soothing irritation, preventing infection and decay, and promoting stronger oral defenses.

- Apply a little clove oil directly to the affected area, or mix a drop in 1 teaspoon of coconut oil for oil pulling.

- Using clove mouthwash twice daily for 5 days cut ventilator pneumonia risk by 50% vs. standard mouthwash.[160]

- For a potent mouth rinse, boil 1 teaspoon of whole cloves in water, strain, and use as a rinse twice daily for freshness, protection, and relief.

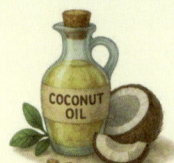

Coconut Oil

Coconut oil's lauric acid gives it antimicrobial properties that reduce harmful oral bacteria. Regular oil pulling helps decrease plaque, soothe and protect sensitive gums, freshen breath, reduce inflammation, and support overall oral health naturally and effectively, enhancing hygiene and preventing future issues.

- Use 1 tablespoon of coconut oil for oil pulling, swishing for 10-15 minutes before spitting it out, daily.

- Oil pulling with coconut oil can significantly reduce plaque index scores and salivary bacterial colony counts.[161]

- Start with shorter sessions (3-5 minutes) if new to oil pulling, gradually building up to 10-15 minutes.

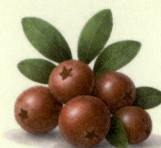

Cranberry

Cranberries contain proanthocyanidins that inhibit bacteria from sticking to teeth and gums, helping to prevent plaque formation. Their antioxidant properties further support gum health by reducing inflammation, preventing oxidative damage, and promoting a cleaner, healthier oral environment.

- Drink 4 oz of unsweetened cranberry juice daily.

- Cranberry polyphenols can inhibit up to 95% of dental plaque formation.[162]

- Use unsweetened cranberry juice to avoid added sugars. For a flavor twist, mix with a splash of lemon juice and enjoy chilled for extra refreshment.

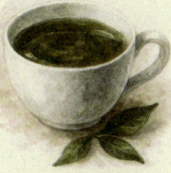

Achieve a healthy smile – explore natural ways to protect teeth and gums, preventing issues and enhancing overall oral health.

Green Tea

Green tea is rich in catechins, powerful antioxidants that inhibit oral bacteria growth and reduce inflammation. Regular use helps strengthen gum tissue, prevent plaque buildup, reduce bad breath, and support long-term gum and overall oral health.

- Drink 1-2 cups of unsweetened green tea daily, or use as a rinse after steeping.

- Long-term green tea use raised the chances of keeping 20+ teeth by 37.7% in older men.[163]

- Opt for freshly brewed green tea instead of bottled versions for higher catechin content.

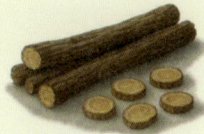

Licorice Root

Licorice root contains glycyrrhizin, an anti-inflammatory and antibacterial compound that helps prevent plaque buildup and soothes irritated gums. It's also beneficial for preventing cavities due to its antimicrobial effects, supporting a healthier mouth and fresher breath.

- Use a licorice root stick to gently massage gums, or use licorice tea as a mouth rinse.

- Compounds in licorice root effectively killed two major bacteria responsible for dental cavities and gum disease.[164]

- Avoid commercial licorice candy, as it doesn't have the same active compounds as natural licorice root.

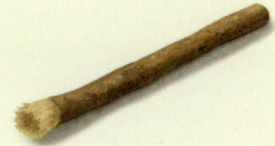

Miswak

Miswak contains antibacterial compounds that help prevent plaque, reduce gum inflammation, and strengthen teeth. It acts as both a toothbrush and toothpaste, helping clean the teeth while releasing ingredients that fight bacteria and freshen breath.

- Chew the frayed end of a miswak stick for ~2 minutes, then use it like a brush on all tooth surfaces daily.

- Miswak sticks and Miswak toothbrushes reduced plaque and gingivitis as effectively as standard brushes over three weeks.[165]

- Soak a new miswak stick in water for a few hours before first use to soften the fibers, enhance flexibility, and ensure gentle, effective cleaning.

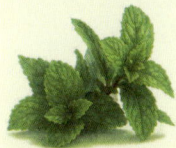

Peppermint

Peppermint contains menthol, which has antibacterial properties that fight bad breath and reduce harmful mouth bacteria. Its natural cooling effect soothes gum irritation, promotes a clean feeling, and helps keep your mouth fresh—so you can feel confident about your breath, naturally and without harsh chemicals.

- Brew peppermint tea and use it as a mouth rinse, or chew on fresh peppermint leaves.

- Peppermint mouth rinse improved bad breath symptoms in 50% of participants after one week.[166]

- For enhanced benefits, pair peppermint with green tea for a powerful antibacterial mouth rinse that freshens breath.

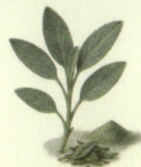

Sage

Sage has powerful anti-inflammatory and antimicrobial properties that help reduce gum swelling and inhibit bacterial growth in the mouth. It is effective for maintaining healthy gums, soothing irritation, preventing oral infections and bad breath, and promoting long-term oral wellness, freshness, and resilience.

- Brew sage tea and use as a mouth rinse twice daily, or gently rub a sage leaf on your gums.

- Using sage mouthwash can reduce cavity-causing bacteria in dental plaque by 92%.[167]

- Add a pinch of salt to the rinse to boost its antibacterial power, help clean more effectively, and support healing in your mouth.

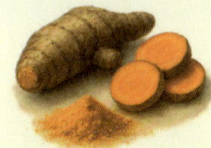

Turmeric

Turmeric contains curcumin, a powerful anti-inflammatory and antimicrobial compound that helps reduce gum swelling, fight infection, and promote healing. It's especially beneficial for treating inflamed or bleeding gums and supporting overall oral health, freshness, gum resilience, and long-term dental wellness.

- Mix 1 teaspoon turmeric with water to form a paste, apply to gums, leave briefly, then rinse with water.

- Turmeric significantly reduced oral mucositis severity in head and neck cancer patients, after six weeks.[168]

- Pair with black pepper to increase curcumin absorption, enhancing its effectiveness, anti-inflammatory benefits, and overall healing potential.

Gum Health & Inflammation

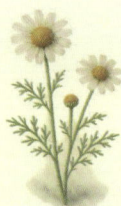

Chamomile

Chamomile has anti-inflammatory and antimicrobial properties that help reduce gum swelling and prevent infection, supporting overall gum and oral tissue health, and soothing irritation of sensitive areas.

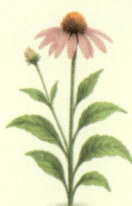

Echinacea

Echinacea supports gum health by boosting the immune response and reducing inflammation. It may help prevent and manage gum infections and promote healing.

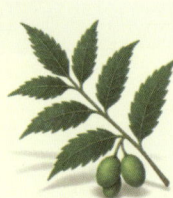

Neem

Neem is known for its strong antibacterial effects. It targets harmful oral bacteria, reduces gum inflammation, prevents plaque buildup, and is used in gum care for maintaining healthy teeth and gums.

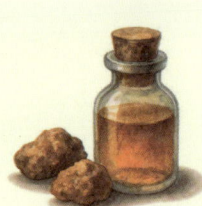

Myrrh

Myrrh acts as an astringent that strengthens gum tissue and reduces inflammation. Its antiseptic properties also help protect against gum infections, promote healing, and support overall oral health.

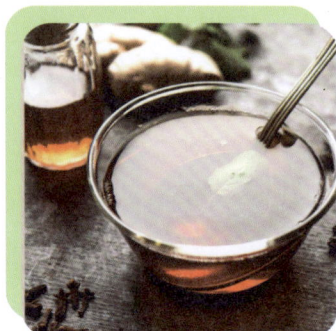

Anti-Inflammatory Clove & Sage Mouth Rinse

This powerful rinse combines clove, known for its anti-inflammatory and antimicrobial effects, with sage, a soothing herb that helps reduce gum swelling and fight bacteria. Perfect for reducing inflammation and promoting healthier gums.

Ingredients:
- 1 cup water
- 1 tsp dried sage leaves
- 1/2 tsp ground clove or 4 whole cloves
- Optional: 1 tsp salt

Instructions:
1. Boil the water and add the sage and cloves.
2. Let it simmer for 5 minutes, then cool and strain.
3. Rinse your mouth with this solution twice daily, swishing for 30 seconds before spitting it out.

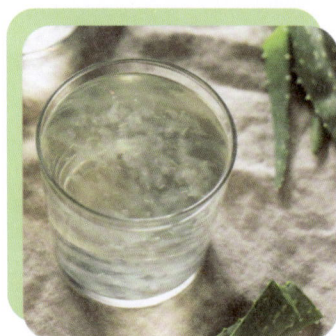

Aloe Vera & Peppermint Gum Soother

Aloe vera is renowned for its healing and anti-inflammatory properties, while peppermint offers a refreshing taste and additional antibacterial support. This gum soother can calm inflammation and freshen breath.

Ingredients:
- 1 tbsp aloe vera gel
- 1/2 cup water
- 3-4 drops peppermint essential oil

Instructions:
1. Mix the aloe vera gel, water, and peppermint oil until combined.
2. Swish the mixture in your mouth for 1-2 minutes, focusing on the gum area.
3. Use once a day for soothing relief.

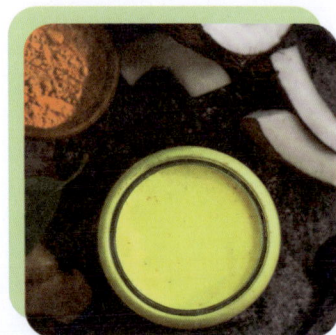

Coconut Oil & Turmeric Gum Massage Paste

Combining coconut oil's natural antibacterial qualities with turmeric's anti-inflammatory power, this paste provides gentle relief for inflamed gums while helping to prevent plaque buildup.

Ingredients:
- 1 tbsp coconut oil
- 1/2 tsp turmeric powder

Instructions:
1. Mix coconut oil and turmeric until you form a smooth paste.
2. Apply the paste to your gums and massage gently for 1-2 minutes.
3. Let it sit for 5 minutes, then rinse with warm water. Use 2-3 times weekly for best results.

Tooth Health & Sensitivity

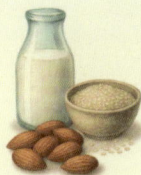

Calcium-Rich Foods

Foods high in calcium help strengthen tooth enamel and reduce sensitivity. They protect against decay by supporting the structural integrity of teeth, and maintaining dental health.

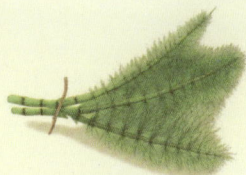

Horsetail

Horsetail is rich in silica, a mineral that reinforces tooth enamel. It helps reduce sensitivity by improving mineral density, supporting dental strength, and promoting long-term oral resilience.

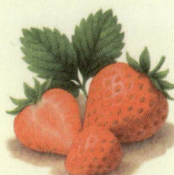

Strawberry

Strawberries contain malic acid and antioxidants that support natural tooth whitening. They help strengthen enamel, reduce surface stains, and brighten your smile without increasing sensitivity.

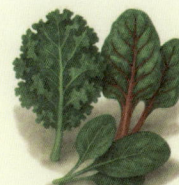

Vitamin K-Rich Foods

Vitamin K is essential for enamel mineralization and overall tooth health. It helps reduce sensitivity and protects teeth from decay by improving mineral retention.

Baking Soda & Coconut Oil Tooth Polish

This gentle polish uses baking soda for a mild abrasive effect that cleans and whitens teeth without damaging enamel. Coconut oil complements by reducing bacteria and protecting sensitive areas.

Ingredients:
- 1 tbsp baking soda
- 1 tbsp coconut oil

Instructions:
1. Mix baking soda and coconut oil into a smooth paste.
2. Apply a small amount to your toothbrush and brush gently in circular motions for 1-2 minutes.
3. Rinse thoroughly with water. Use 1-2 times per week to reduce sensitivity and improve tooth brightness.

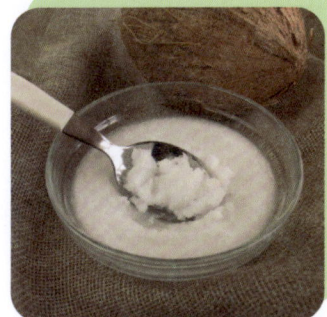

Green Tea & Cranberry Rinse

Green tea contains catechins, which help protect teeth from decay and reduce sensitivity, while cranberry prevents bacteria from sticking to teeth and causing plaque. This rinse also helps to freshen breath naturally.

Ingredients:
- 1 cup brewed green tea (cooled)
- 2 tbsp pure cranberry juice (unsweetened)

Instructions:
1. Combine green tea and cranberry juice.
2. Rinse your mouth with this solution twice daily, swishing for 30 seconds each time.
3. Use regularly to strengthen enamel and reduce tooth sensitivity.

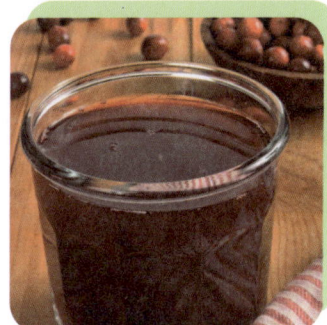

Peppermint & Licorice Root Sensitivity Soother

Peppermint helps freshen breath and reduce oral bacteria, while licorice root (especially DGL) soothes irritated gums and supports a healthy mouth. Together, they create a gentle blend for oral care and overall mouth health.

Ingredients (Serves 1–2):
- 1 tsp dried peppermint leaves (or 1 peppermint tea bag)
- 1 tsp dried licorice root (or 1 licorice tea bag; use DGL if needed for blood pressure sensitivity)
- 1½ cups just-boiled water
- 1 tsp raw honey (optional, for soothing and flavor)

Instructions:
1. In a teapot or mug, combine the peppermint and licorice root.
2. Pour over freshly boiled water and cover.
3. Let steep for 8–10 minutes, then strain if using loose herbs.
4. Stir in honey if desired and sip slowly while warm.

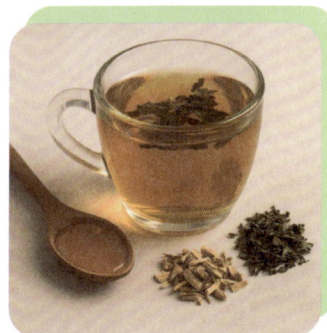

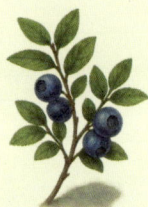

Eye Health

Bilberry

Bilberries contain anthocyanins, powerful antioxidants that help improve blood flow to the retina, enhancing night vision and reducing eye strain from prolonged screen time. Studies also show bilberry's benefits in reducing retinal inflammation and oxidative stress.

Take 1 teaspoon of bilberry extract daily or add fresh bilberries to your diet.

Taking 120–160 mg of bilberry extract daily may ease eye fatigue and dryness from screen use.[169]

Combine with green tea for added antioxidant effects, especially beneficial after long screen exposure.

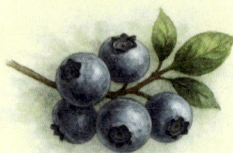

Blueberries

Blueberries are high in antioxidants, particularly anthocyanins, which protect the retina from oxidative stress and support better blood circulation to the eyes. Regular blueberry intake can slow the onset of age-related eye issues, enhancing overall eye health.

Eat 1/2 cup of fresh or frozen blueberries daily.

One weekly serving of blueberries is linked to a 68% lower risk of age-related macular degeneration in women.[170]

For an eye-boosting smoothie, blend banana, blueberries, leafy greens, and almond milk.

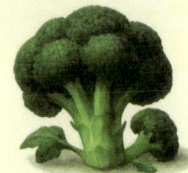

Broccoli

Broccoli is rich in lutein and zeaxanthin, two carotenoids that protect against cataracts and age-related macular degeneration by filtering harmful blue light and reducing oxidative stress. It also contains vitamin C, which supports collagen production, eye health, and vision clarity.

Include 1 cup of steamed or lightly sautéed broccoli in your meals several times a week.

One cup of raw broccoli provides 81.2 mg of vitamin C, covering most daily needs and helping prevent cataracts.[171]

Pair with olive oil or nuts to boost absorption of carotenoids, enhancing their effectiveness for even greater eye health benefits.

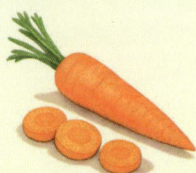

Carrot

Carrots are well-known for their high beta-carotene content, a precursor to vitamin A, which is essential for good vision and particularly important for night vision. Beta-carotene also protects the cornea, supports the eye's natural moisture, and helps prevent dryness, irritation, and overall eye fatigue.

Consume 1/2 cup of raw or lightly cooked carrots daily to maximize beta-carotene intake.

Consuming 1,070 µg RAE of vitamin A from foods like carrots provides 118% of the daily value, supporting normal vision.[172]

Eat with a small amount of fat (like olive oil or nuts) for better absorption of beta-carotene and enhanced nutrient uptake.

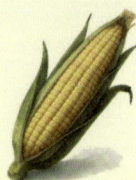

Corn

Corn is a good source of lutein and zeaxanthin, along with vitamin C and antioxidants. These nutrients help filter harmful blue light, protect the retina, and support overall eye health, visual function, and long-term clarity and sharpness—especially as the eyes age naturally and oxidative stress increases.

Eat 1 ear of corn or 1 cup of cooked corn kernels several times per week, boiled or grilled.

One study found that sweet corn extract can help protect eye cells from inflammation, a key cause of age-related sight loss.[173]

Eat corn with a dab of butter or oil and a pinch of salt – the fat helps absorb the lutein more effectively and boosts its benefits.

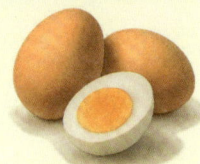

Eggs

Egg yolks are a rich source of lutein and zeaxanthin, powerful antioxidants that accumulate in the retina and help protect the eyes from age-related vision loss, oxidative stress, and damage from harmful light exposure, enhancing overall visual performance, protection, and long-term eye health.

Include 1 whole egg per day (ideally free-range).

Two eggs daily for four months, especially enriched ones, boosted eye nutrients and slightly improved age-related vision health.[174]

Lutein is fat-soluble – cooking eggs with a bit of healthy fat helps your body absorb it better, maximizing its protective benefits for the eyes.

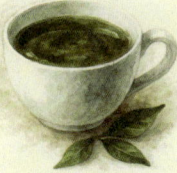

Eye Health

Green Tea

Green tea contains powerful antioxidants, including catechins, which have been shown to protect the eye's delicate tissues from oxidative stress. Its anti-inflammatory properties also help alleviate eye strain and reduce the risk of cataracts and AMD over time.

- Drink 1-2 cups of green tea daily for its protective effects.

- Drinking green tea daily may reduce the risk of developing glaucoma by up to 74%.[175]

- Apply cooled green tea bags over closed eyes for 10 minutes to soothe tired eyes and reduce puffiness.

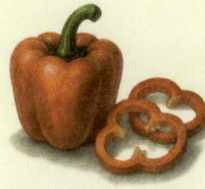

Red Bell Pepper

Red bell peppers are packed with vitamin C and beta-carotene that are both powerful antioxidants that protect the eye's tissues from oxidative damage. The beta-carotene converts to vitamin A, supporting night vision, reducing age-related eye issues, and promoting overall visual health.

- Consume raw in salads or as snacks; aim for 1 cup per day to maximize nutrient intake.

- Consuming red bell peppers regularly may reduce the risk of developing cataracts by up to 25%.[176]

- Enjoy red bell peppers raw, as cooking can significantly reduce their vitamin C content and antioxidant potency.

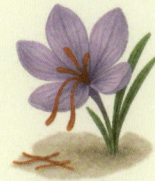

Saffron

Saffron contains crocin and safranal, compounds that protect retinal cells and delay photoreceptor degeneration. It improves light sensitivity, enhances retinal blood flow, and may help slow the progression of age-related macular degeneration.

- Steep 5-10 threads in warm milk or tea and drink daily for maximum benefits.

- Daily saffron improved vision by two Snellen lines after 3 months in people with early age-related macular degeneration.[177]

- Pair saffron with a pinch of black pepper to boost its absorption, enhance its benefits, and maximize its healing potential.

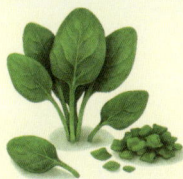

Spinach

Spinach contains lutein and zeaxanthin, antioxidants that accumulate in the retina and lens, acting as a natural filter against harmful blue light. They help reduce eye strain, enhance visual clarity, and delay the onset of cataracts, macular degeneration, and other age-related eye conditions, supporting lifelong vision health.

- Include a handful of raw or lightly steamed spinach in daily meals, smoothies, or salads.

- Consuming spinach daily may reduce the risk of developing age-related macular degeneration by up to 43%.[178]

- Add a splash of olive oil to spinach to enhance the absorption of lutein and zeaxanthin, boosting effectiveness for eye health protection.

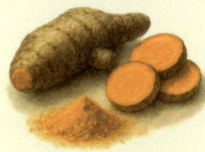

Turmeric

Turmeric contains curcumin, known for its powerful anti-inflammatory and antioxidant effects. Curcumin helps protect the retina and optic nerve, reducing the risk of age-related degeneration and easing symptoms of dry eye, eye strain, and oxidative damage to delicate eye tissues, supporting long-term visual health.

- Take 1/4 to 1/2 teaspoon of turmeric daily with a pinch of black pepper to boost absorption.

- Daily consumption of turmeric may reduce the risk of developing cataracts by up to 25%.[179]

- Mix turmeric with a bit of fat (like coconut or olive oil) to enhance bioavailability and boost absorption efficiency.

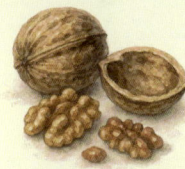

Walnuts

Walnuts are rich in omega-3 fatty acids and vitamin E, both essential for reducing inflammation and maintaining healthy tear production. Omega-3s help protect the retina from oxidative stress, ease eye strain, promote clear vision, and support long-term eye function, comfort, visual clarity, and overall eye health.

- Eat a small handful (about 1 ounce) of walnuts daily as a snack or salad topping.

- Adding walnuts to your diet may reduce age-related macular degeneration risk by up to 25%.[180]

- Soak walnuts overnight to increase nutrient absorption, improve digestion, and reduce bitterness for better taste.

Vision Support & Clarity

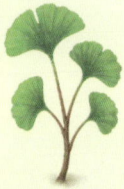

Ginkgo Biloba

Ginkgo biloba contains flavonoid antioxidants that improve blood flow to the retina. It may support visual function and help protect overall eye health.

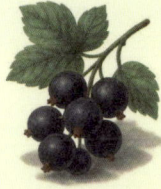

Black Currants

Black currants are rich in anthocyanins, which enhance blood circulation to the eyes. They may improve visual sharpness and contrast, reduce eye fatigue, and support retinal function.

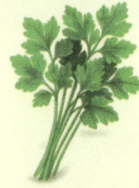

Parsley

Parsley provides lutein and zeaxanthin—carotenoids that protect the eyes from light damage and support visual clarity, eye comfort, and long-term eye function.

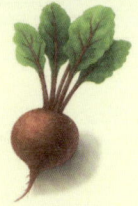

Beetroot

Beetroot contains natural nitrates that boost blood flow and oxygen delivery to the eyes. This may support sharper vision, reduce eye fatigue, and help protect against age-related decline.

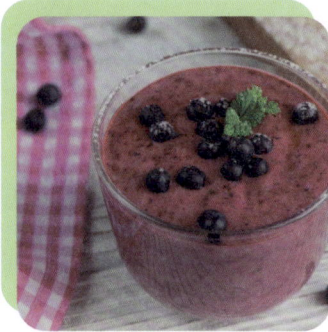

Bilberry & Blueberry Antioxidant Smoothie

Bilberries and blueberries are packed with anthocyanins, potent antioxidants known to improve blood flow to the eyes and protect the retina from oxidative stress. Paired with almonds, which contain vitamin E, this smoothie supports long-term eye health and visual clarity.

Ingredients:
- 1/2 cup bilberries or bilberry powder
- 1/2 cup fresh blueberries
- 1 tbsp almond butter (or 5-6 almonds, soaked overnight)
- 1 cup unsweetened almond milk
- 1/2 tsp honey (optional)

Instructions:
1. Add all ingredients to a blender.
2. Blend until smooth and creamy.
3. Pour into a glass and enjoy as a morning or midday boost for eye health.

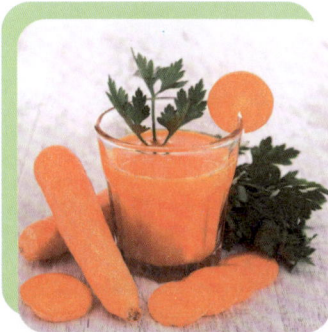

Carrot & Parsley Juice Blend

Carrots are rich in beta-carotene, a precursor of vitamin A essential for vision, while parsley is loaded with lutein and zeaxanthin, which protect against harmful light exposure and improve visual performance.

Ingredients:
- 2 large carrots, peeled and chopped
- 1/2 cup fresh parsley leaves
- 1/2 lemon, juiced
- 1 cup water or coconut water (optional for extra hydration)

Instructions:
1. Add carrots, parsley, and water to a blender, and blend until smooth.
2. Strain the mixture through a sieve or cheesecloth for a smoother juice.
3. Add lemon juice, stir, and drink immediately for the freshest nutrients.

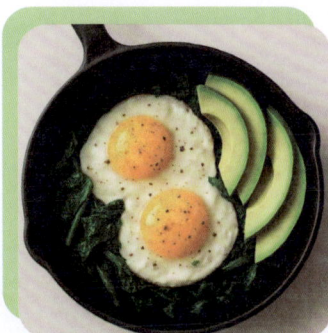

Spinach & Egg Eye Health Skillet

Egg yolks and spinach are rich in lutein and zeaxanthin—key antioxidants that protect the eyes from blue light and AMD. Spinach also adds vitamin C, beta-carotene, and folate for overall eye and vessel health, making this a vision-supportive duo.

Ingredients (Serves 1–2):
- 2 eggs
- 1 cup fresh spinach, roughly chopped
- 1 tsp olive oil or ghee
- Salt and black pepper to taste
- Optional: pinch of turmeric (for extra antioxidant support)
- Optional toppings: Avocado slices, or grated carrot

Instructions:
1. Heat oil in a skillet; sauté spinach for 1–2 mins.
2. Crack eggs over spinach, cover, and cook 3–4 mins.
3. Season with salt, pepper, and optional turmeric.
4. Serve with veggies or whole grain toast.

Age-Related Eye Conditions

EXTRA HERBS

Eyebright

Eyebright has long been used to ease eye strain, redness, and irritation. It contains compounds that support comfort during prolonged screen time and visual fatigue.

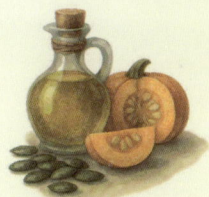

Pumpkin Seeds

Pumpkin seeds are rich in zinc and vitamin E, which support retinal health and may help reduce the risk of age-related macular degeneration, while also protecting and maintaining clear vision.

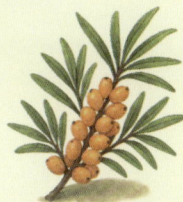

Sea Buckthorn

Sea buckthorn is high in antioxidants and fatty acids that support eye hydration and maintain the moisture barrier. It helps protect against oxidative stress, and guards against age-related eye conditions.

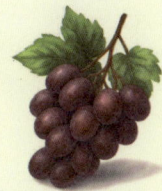

Red Grapes

Red grapes contain resveratrol and other antioxidants that protect retinal cells from damage. They may help reduce oxidative stress, support healthy blood vessels in the eyes, and lower the risk of AMD.

Broccoli & Red Pepper Vision Boost Soup

Broccoli and red bell pepper are both rich in vitamins C and E, essential for protecting eye cells from free radical damage and supporting the prevention of age-related vision decline.

Ingredients:
- 1/2 cup broccoli florets
- 1/2 red bell pepper, chopped
- 1 small carrot, chopped
- 1 1/2 cups vegetable broth
- Salt and pepper to taste

Instructions:
1. In a small pot, add vegetable broth, broccoli, red bell pepper, and carrot.
2. Bring to a boil, then reduce to a simmer and cook until vegetables are tender (about 10-15 minutes).
3. Blend the soup until smooth, season with salt and pepper to taste, and enjoy warm as a nourishing, eye-supporting meal.

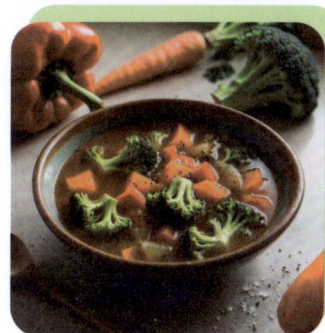

Eyebright & Red Grape Tea

Eyebright has traditionally been used to soothe eye strain and support overall eye health. Red grapes add antioxidants that help protect the eye tissue from aging.

Ingredients:
- 1 tsp dried eyebright
- 1/2 cup fresh red grapes, halved
- 1 cup boiling water
- 1 tsp honey (optional)

Instructions:
1. Place eyebright and grapes in a cup.
2. Pour boiling water over the ingredients and let steep for 5 minutes.
3. Strain, add honey if desired, and enjoy warm.

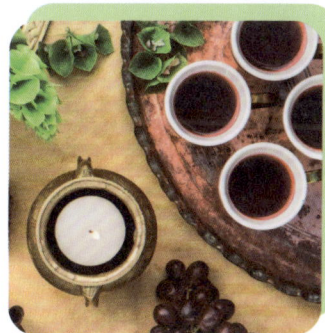

Sea Buckthorn & Ginger Eye Health Tonic

Sea buckthorn is loaded with omega-7 fatty acids, known for supporting skin and eye tissue health, while ginger helps improve blood circulation, reducing strain and inflammation around the eyes.

Ingredients:
- 1 tsp sea buckthorn oil or juice
- 1/2 tsp fresh ginger, grated
- 1 cup warm water
- 1/2 tsp honey (optional, for taste)

Instructions:
1. In a cup, combine the sea buckthorn oil, grated ginger, and warm water.
2. Stir well, and add honey if desired.
3. Sip slowly and enjoy the soothing effects on the eyes and body. This tonic can be consumed once daily.

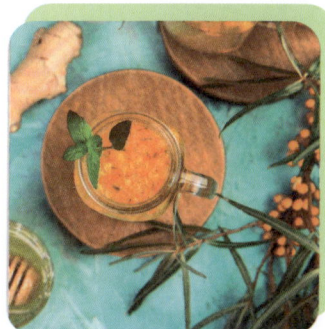

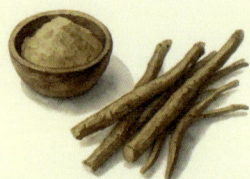

Men's Health

Support your vitality – learn how natural remedies can enhance energy, stamina, and overall wellness for men.

Ashwagandha

Ashwagandha helps lower cortisol (stress hormone), and can help improve testosterone levels. It is also found to boost testosterone directly, improve sperm quality, enhance muscle strength and recovery, and support energy, mood, endurance, and overall vitality.

- 500–600 mg per day of a high-concentration root extract is a typical effective dose.

- One study in infertile men found ashwagandha supplementation led to a 15% jump in testosterone.[181]

- Take it in the evening, as it also aids relaxation and sleep — and better sleep itself can help boost testosterone naturally.

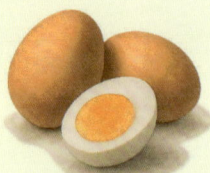

Eggs

Eggs are often called "nature's multivitamin" for good reason – they are packed with high-quality protein, healthy fats, and essential micronutrients. Each egg provides about 6–7 g of complete protein, aiding in muscle building, repair, hormone production, and overall vitality.

- 1 egg per day is a common guideline, but many healthy men can eat 2–3 eggs a day.

- Resistance-trained men had more muscle protein synthesis eating whole eggs post-workout than egg whites with equal protein.[182]

- Don't toss the yolk! The yolk contains most of the vitamins (A, D, B12, etc.), minerals, and essential fats.

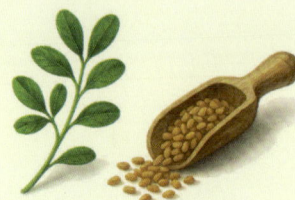

Fenugreek

Fenugreek contains natural compounds that may help boost testosterone levels or increase its availability in the body. It has been shown and improve libido and sexual performance, support healthy energy levels, and may also aid in muscle strength, endurance, and recovery.

- Soak 1–2 teaspoons of seeds overnight, or take 1–2 teaspoons of powder or 300–600 mg fenugreek extract daily.

- In 12 weeks, fenugreek raised free testosterone by 46% in older men, and improved morning erections and sexual frequency.[183]

- If you cook with fenugreek seeds, dry-toast them first to reduce bitterness, then grind them for better flavor and easier digestion.

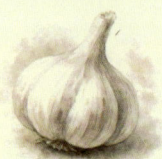

Garlic

Garlic contains compounds (like allicin, formed when garlic is crushed) that improve blood pressure and circulation. This helps reduce strain on the heart and can enhance blood flow to muscles and genital organs, supporting erectile function, stamina, overall cardiovascular health, energy levels, and physical performance.

- Aim for 1–2 cloves of fresh garlic per day.

- Garlic supplements lowered BP by ~3.7/3.4 mmHg (systolic/diastolic) in a meta-analysis of 17 trials.[184]

- Crush or chop garlic and let it sit for 10 minutes to allow allicin, its key compound, to fully form and maximize its health benefits.

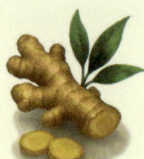

Ginger

Ginger is rich in antioxidants and helps reduce inflammation, protecting the body's cells, including sperm cells. It also improves blood flow by relaxing blood vessels, may slightly lower blood pressure, and supports reproductive health, cardiovascular function, overall vitality, hormonal balance, and sexual performance.

- Take 1–2 g ginger daily—about ½ teaspoon powder or a 1-inch piece of fresh root.

- In infertile men, 3 months of ginger boosted sperm count, motility, morphology, and testosterone levels significantly.[185]

- You can add ginger powder to smoothies or oatmeal (it pairs well with cinnamon) for extra flavor, warmth, and health benefits.

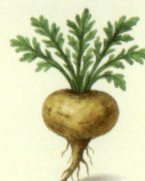

Maca

Maca root is a natural libido booster and fertility enhancer. While it doesn't directly raise testosterone, it supports sexual health through hormonal balance, improves energy levels, and enhances overall stamina, endurance, well-being, mood, focus, physical performance, and reproductive vitality.

- 1.5 to 3 g of maca root powder per day is the typical dose range.

- Men who took 1,500–3,000 mg of maca daily reported a significant increase in sexual desire after eight weeks vs. a placebo.[186]

- Try adding maca to your coffee — it has a malty, slightly sweet taste and blends well for a nutritious energy boost.

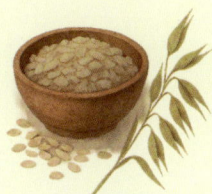

Oats

Oats are a heart-healthy grain rich in beta-glucan, which helps lower LDL (bad) cholesterol and improve circulation. They also provide magnesium and arginine, which support healthy blood vessels and hormonal balance while stabilizing blood sugar levels naturally.

🍽 One bowl of oatmeal (¾–1 cup dry oats) daily provides 3 g of beta-glucan for blood sugar support.

⚗ A meta-analysis found that consuming 3 g of oat beta-glucan daily reduced cholesterol by roughly 8-10%.[187]

🌿 Choose minimally processed oats (old-fashioned or steel-cut) over instant oats to maximize fiber and keep the glycemic index lower.

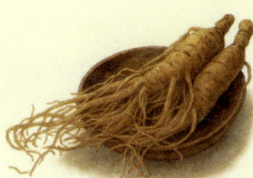

Panax Ginseng (Asian Ginseng)

Panax ginseng is an adaptogen that fights fatigue, boosts circulation, and improves sexual function and libido. It may also support testosterone through effects on the hypothalamus-pituitary-testicular axis and reduce oxidative stress.

🍽 200–400 mg of a standardized Panax ginseng extract, 1–3 times per day.

⚗ Korean red ginseng (900 mg, 3x/day) improved erectile function, with 60% reporting better erections and rigidity.[188]

🌿 Take ginseng earlier in the day, as it can be stimulating and may interfere with sleep if taken too late in the evening.

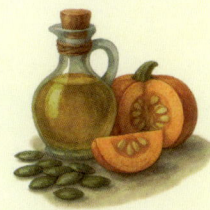

Pumpkin Seeds

Pumpkin seeds are an excellent source of zinc – a mineral essential for normal prostate function and testosterone production. They also contain antioxidants and healthy fats that support heart health and circulation, while reducing inflammation and boosting immune defense.

🍽 Aim for a handful of seeds (1–2 ounces) per day for general benefits.

⚗ In men with benign prostatic hyperplasia, pumpkin seed treatment significantly reduced urinary symptoms compared to placebo.[189]

🌿 Soak raw seeds overnight and then dry them to reduce phytic acid, enhance digestion, and improve mineral absorption and bioavailability.

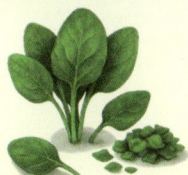

Spinach

Spinach and other dark leafy greens are high in magnesium, which supports testosterone production and muscle function. They also contain natural nitrates that boost blood flow, aiding in healthy blood pressure, improved exercise performance, enhanced erectile function, stamina, endurance, and overall vitality.

🍽 Include at least 1 cup of spinach (or other leafy greens) every day or most days.

⚗ Taking 2 g of spinach extract daily for 12 weeks plus exercise improved muscle strength more than exercise alone.[190]

🌿 Lightly cook your spinach to increase the availability of certain nutrients and reduce oxalates, which can interfere with mineral absorption.

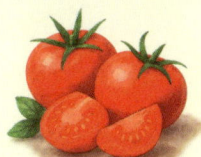

Tomatoes

Tomatoes are high in lycopene, a powerful antioxidant that accumulates in areas like the prostate. It helps reduce oxidative damage and inflammation, which can lower the risk of prostate problems. Lycopene may also protect sperm, support male fertility, promote overall reproductive health, and enhance hormonal balance.

🍽 Aim for 10–15 mg of lycopene daily—about ½–1 cup cooked tomato sauce or 6–10 raw tomatoes weekly.

⚗ In healthy young men, 14 mg of lycopene daily for 12 weeks improved sperm motility and morphology.[191]

🌿 Cook your tomatoes with a bit of fat (like olive oil) to maximize lycopene absorption and enhance its antioxidant benefits.

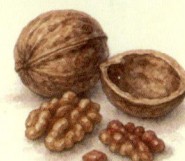

Walnuts

Nuts are rich in arginine, a nutrient that helps the body produce nitric oxide, which relaxes blood vessels and improves blood flow. This enhanced circulation supports healthy erections, boosts sexual arousal and libido, and contributes to overall cardiovascular, reproductive, hormonal health, vitality, and performance.

🍽 Aim for a variety of unsalted, unroasted nuts in moderation (1–2 ounces daily).

⚗ In older men, 15 g of walnuts daily for 6 weeks improved testosterone, cholesterol, cortisol, and inflammation.[192]

🌿 Keep mixed nuts on hand for a healthy, energizing snack that supports daily nutrition and well-being.

Prostate Health

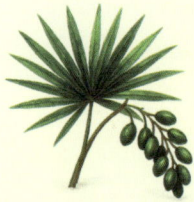

Saw Palmetto (Serenoa repens)

Saw palmetto helps block DHT, the hormone linked to prostate growth. It may reduce prostate size, improve urine flow, and ease symptoms like frequent urination and a weak stream.

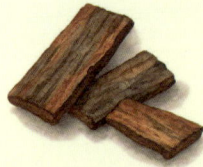

Pygeum (African Plum Tree Bark)

Pygeum supports prostate health by reducing swelling and balancing hormones. It can help improve urine flow, reduce inflammation, and support better bladder emptying.

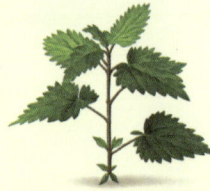

Stinging Nettle Root

Nettle root may lower DHT and estrogen levels while supporting free testosterone. It helps ease urinary symptoms such as weak flow, urgency, and frequent nighttime urination.

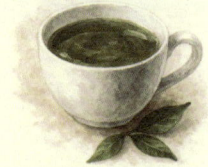

Green Tea

Green tea is rich in antioxidants that protect prostate cells and reduce inflammation. It may slow prostate growth, improve urine flow, support healthy PSA levels, and enhance hormonal balance and wellness.

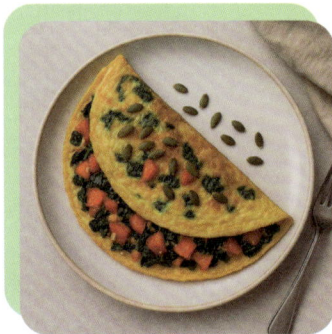

Spinach & Tomato Power Omelette with Garlic

This omelette is good for prostate health because tomatoes have lycopene, which may protect cells; spinach adds zinc and folate for hormone balance; and garlic fights inflammation, all supporting a healthier prostate.

Ingredients (2 servings):

- 4 whole eggs
- 1 cup fresh spinach leaves, chopped
- 1 small tomato, diced
- 2 cloves garlic, minced
- 1 tbsp extra-virgin olive oil
- Salt and pepper to taste

Instructions:

1. Beat eggs with salt and pepper.
2. Sauté garlic in oil for 30 secs.
3. Add tomato and spinach; cook 1–2 mins.
4. Pour in eggs, cook 30 secs, then lift edges to let egg flow.
5. Fold and cook 1 more min.
6. Serve warm, topped with seeds or yogurt if desired.

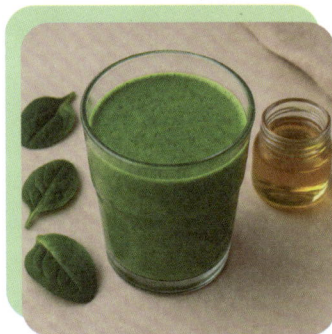

Green Men's Health Smoothie

This smoothie is great for men's health because spinach supports prostate and heart health with vitamins and antioxidants, maca boosts testosterone and libido, and ginger improves circulation, reduces inflammation, and supports hormone balance naturally.

Ingredients (1 large smoothie):

- 1 cup kefir or Greek yogurt
- 1 cup spinach (or ½ cup frozen)
- 1 small banana
- 1 tsp maca powder
- 1-inch piece fresh ginger
- 1 tbsp nut butter
- ¼ cup water or ice cubes
- Optional: 1 tsp ashwagandha, 1 tbsp raw cacao

Instructions:

1. Add all ingredients to a blender.
2. Blend on high until smooth and creamy.
3. Adjust thickness with water or ice as needed.
4. Taste and add honey if desired. Serve immediately.

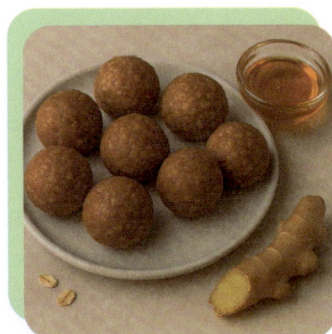

Pumpkin Seed & Ginger Energy Bites

These energy bites are good for prostate health because pumpkin seeds are rich in zinc, which supports prostate function and hormone balance, while ginger reduces inflammation and may help protect against prostate cell damage.

Ingredients (makes ~12 bites):

- 1 cup rolled oats
- ½ cup natural nut butter
- ⅓ cup chopped pumpkin seeds
- 2 tbsp maca powder (optional)
- 2 tbsp honey
- 1 tbsp minced fresh ginger (or 1 tsp powder)
- 1 tsp ground fenugreek (optional)
- Pinch of salt

Instructions:

1. Mix oats, seeds, maca, fenugreek, and salt.
2. Add nut butter, honey, and ginger; mix well.
3. Adjust texture with water or oats if needed.
4. Roll into balls and chill for 30 mins.
5. Store in the fridge for up to 1 week.

Testosterone & Sexual Function

EXTRA HERBS

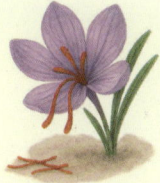

Saffron

Saffron contains crocin and safranal, which reduce oxidative stress and support hormone production. It may enhance libido by boosting dopamine and improving blood flow to reproductive organs.

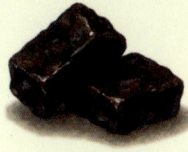

Shilajit

Shilajit is rich in fulvic acid and minerals that support testosterone and DHEA levels. It may improve energy, sperm count, and motility, supporting male fertility and reproductive health.

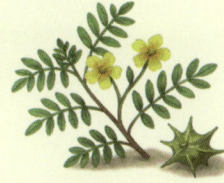

Tribulus Terrestris

Tribulus contains compounds that may raise LH and support testosterone production. It also promotes better blood flow, which can enhance erectile function and overall sexual performance.

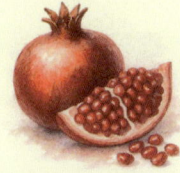

Pomegranate

Pomegranate juice is high in antioxidants like punicalagins, which protect testosterone-producing cells and sperm. It also boosts nitric oxide, improving blood flow and erectile health.

Ashwagandha "Golden Milk" Nightcap

This nightcap is good for men's overall health because ashwagandha helps reduce stress and boost testosterone, turmeric and ginger fight inflammation, black pepper enhances absorption, and honey and cinnamon support immunity and blood sugar balance.

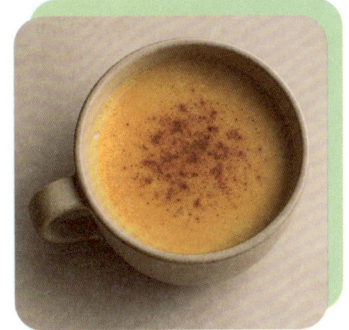

Ingredients (1 serving):

- 1 cup milk of choice
- 1 tsp ashwagandha powder
- ½ tsp turmeric powder (optional)
- ½ tsp ginger powder (or fresh grated)
- Pinch of black pepper
- 1 tsp honey
- ¼ tsp cinnamon (optional)

Instructions:

1. Whisk all ingredients (except honey) into milk in a saucepan.
2. Warm gently over medium-low heat for 3–5 minutes (do not boil).
3. Remove from heat. Stir in honey.
4. Pour into a mug and sip warm 30–60 minutes before bedtime.

Pumpkin Seed & Maca Overnight Oats

This overnight oats recipe is good for testosterone and sexual function because pumpkin seeds provide zinc for testosterone production, and maca root supports libido, energy, and hormonal balance, naturally enhancing sexual health and vitality.

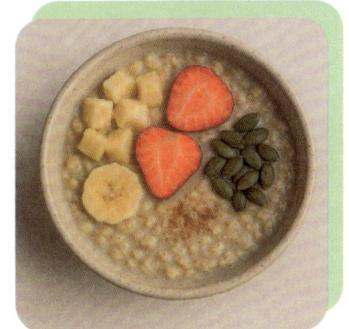

Ingredients (1 serving):

- ½ cup rolled oats
- ¾ cup milk of choice
- ¼ cup Greek yogurt
- 2 tbsp pumpkin seeds
- 1 tsp maca powder
- ½ tsp cinnamon (optional)
- 1–2 tsp honey or maple syrup (optional)
- ¼ cup chopped fruit (e.g., berries or banana)

Instructions:

1. Mix oats, milk, yogurt, maca, and cinnamon.
2. Stir in pumpkin seeds and sweetener.
3. Cover and chill overnight.
4. In the morning, stir, top with fruit, and adjust texture with milk if needed.
5. Enjoy cold or warm.

Fenugreek-Spiced Chicken & Spinach Curry

This curry is good for testosterone and sexual health because fenugreek may naturally boost testosterone levels and libido, while spinach provides magnesium and zinc for hormone balance and improved blood flow, supporting overall sexual function.

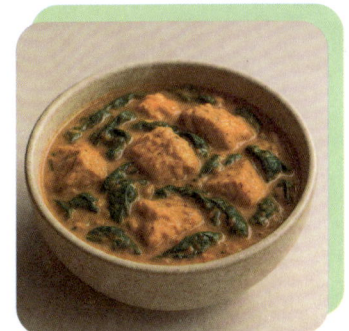

Ingredients (4 servings):

- 1 lb chicken or 1 can chickpeas
- 4 cups fresh (or 1 cup frozen) spinach
- 1 onion, diced
- 3 garlic cloves, minced
- 1 tbsp minced ginger
- 2 tomatoes or 1 cup canned
- 1 cup Greek yogurt
- 2 tbsp olive oil or ghee
- 1 tsp each: fenugreek, cumin, turmeric, coriander
- ½ tsp garam masala or curry powder
- 1 tsp salt, ½ tsp pepper

Instructions:

1. Toast fenugreek and cumin seeds; set aside.
2. Sauté onion in oil, then add garlic and ginger.
3. Stir in spices and toasted seeds.
4. Add chicken; cook 5–7 mins (add chickpeas later if using).
5. Add tomatoes; cook 3–4 mins into a sauce.
6. Lower heat, stir in yogurt.
7. Simmer 5 mins, then add spinach to wilt.
8. Season and simmer 2–3 more mins.
9. Serve with rice or alone.

Kidney Health

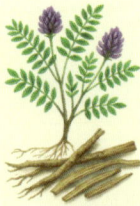

Astragalus

Astragalus may support kidney health by reducing inflammation and oxidative stress, and by improving protein filtration, especially helpful in chronic kidney disease. It also has immune-boosting and anti-inflammatory effects, and may promote vitality and long-term organ function.

🍽 Aim for 9 to 30 g of dried root daily (as tea or decoction), or 250–500 mg extract, 2–3 times daily.

⚗ In diabetic kidney disease, astragalus protected kidney function and reduced urinary protein compared to no treatment.[193]

🌿 Astragalus is available as dried slices – you can simmer a few slices in soups or teas.

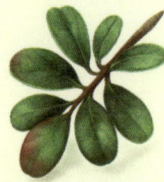

Bearberry Leaf

Uva ursi (also known as bearberry) is a traditional herb used to support urinary health. It contains arbutin, which converts into a natural antibacterial compound in urine, especially when the urine is less acidic. It may help reduce infection risk, soothe irritation, and support overall bladder function.

🍽 Uva ursi is often taken as a tea or capsule at doses around 400–800 mg of extract 2–3 times daily.

⚗ In women with recurrent UTIs, uva-ursi reduced recurrences to 5% vs. 27% with placebo over one year.[194]

🌿 It's not for long-term continuous use due to potential liver toxicity; use for a week or two at a time when needed.

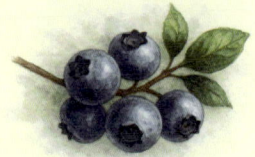

Blueberries

Blueberries are rich in anthocyanins and powerful antioxidants that help reduce oxidative stress and inflammation. These compounds protect kidney tissue from damage, support blood flow, and may lower the risk of chronic kidney disease.

🍽 Aim for ½ to 1 cup (approximately 75–150 g) of blueberries per day.

⚗ Animals with metabolic syndrome given blueberries had much less kidney damage and leaking of protein into their urine vs. placebo.[195]

🌿 Add fresh or frozen blueberries to oatmeal, yogurt, or smoothies for a boost of antioxidants, flavor, and natural sweetness.

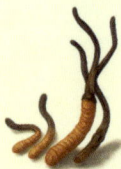

Cordyceps Mushroom

This unique fungus has anti-inflammatory anti-inflammatory and antioxidant properties that help protect kidney cells from damage. It may improve kidney function, reduce protein in the urine, support overall kidney performance, enhance detoxification, reduce inflammation, and promote long-term renal health naturally.

🍽 Typically 3–5 g of mushroom powder or ~1,000 mg of extract daily.

⚗ A review of 22 studies found cordyceps improved kidney function by lowering creatinine, proteinuria, and symptoms.[196]

🌿 Cordyceps is a unique fungus with anti-inflammatory and antioxidant properties that help protect kidney cells from damage.

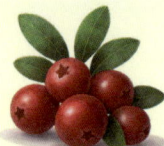

Cranberry

Cranberries contain proanthocyanidins, natural compounds that help prevent harmful bacteria like *E. coli* from sticking to the walls of the bladder and urinary tract. This reduces the risk of infections like UTIs and supports overall urinary tract health, bladder function, immune defense, and natural cleansing processes.

🍽 For UTI prevention, drink 8–10 oz (240–300 ml) of pure cranberry juice daily.

⚗ A Cochrane review of over 50 studies found that cranberry reduced UTI risk by 30–40% in various groups.[197]

🌿 Use unsweetened 100% cranberry juice for maximum benefits. You can dilute it with water if you find it too tart or strong.

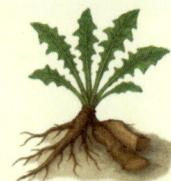

Dandelion Root

Dandelion root is a traditional herbal diuretic and detoxifier. It increases urine production, helping to flush excess fluid and toxins from the kidneys. Dandelion is also rich in antioxidants that reduce cell damage, support liver function, fight inflammation, and promote overall urinary wellness.

🍽 Drink 1–3 cups of tea per day, made from 2–3 teaspoons of dried root simmered for 10–15 minutes.

⚗ A study showed volunteers taking dandelion extract had significantly increased urination within 5 hours.[198]

🌿 Use tea as a natural detox, especially during periods of fluid retention, to help flush out excess water and support kidney function.

Kidney Health

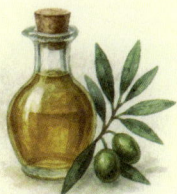

Extra Virgin Olive Oil

Extra-virgin olive oil is rich in polyphenols and monounsaturated fats. Its powerful antioxidants and anti-inflammatory compounds support blood vessel health, reduce oxidative stress, and may improve kidney function markers and overall cardiovascular well-being.

- Aim for 2–4 tablespoons (30–60 ml) daily.

- Patients with kidney disease who consumed olive oil for 9 weeks had lower creatinine and urinary protein.[199]

- Avoid high heat cooking—use oils raw in dressings or drizzle over meals to preserve their nutrients and health benefits.

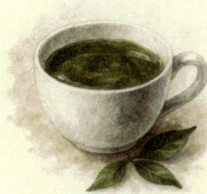

Green Tea

Green tea is rich in antioxidants like catechins, which help reduce inflammation and oxidative stress that can damage the kidneys. It may also support healthy blood pressure and improve kidney function by reducing the risk of kidney-related diseases.

- Aim for 2–3 cups of green tea daily.

- A genetic study found each daily cup of tea cut kidney disease risk by 20% and improved function.[200]

- Brew at 175°F (80°C) for 2–3 minutes to avoid bitterness and preserve the tea's delicate flavor and health benefits.

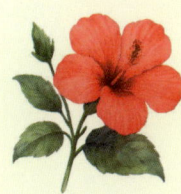

Hibiscus

Hibiscus helps protect the kidneys from damage and keeps them working properly. It has natural antioxidants that reduce swelling and stress in the kidneys. Studies show it can lower harmful markers like creatinine and urea, especially when the kidneys are under stress from drugs or illness.

- Aim for 1–2 cups of tea daily (1.25 – 2 g dried calyx per cup) or 100–250 mg extract.

- Hibiscus reduced kidney damage markers like urea and creatinine, showing protection, especially in drug-induced kidney injury.[201]

- Enjoy hibiscus as a tangy tea— served hot or iced—for a refreshing drink rich in antioxidants and heart-supportive benefits.

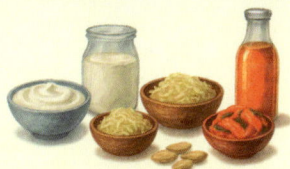

Probiotics (Lactobacillus)

Beneficial bacteria, especially certain *Lactobacillus* strains, can help maintain a healthy urinary tract by preventing harmful bacteria from colonizing. Recurrent UTIs often relate to a disrupted vaginal microbiome (in women) or gut microbiome.

- Use probiotic-rich foods or supplements with *Lactobacillus rhamnosus GR-1* and *L. reuteri RC-14*.

- One study found that both cranberry–lingonberry juice and a *Lactobacillus* drink helped reduce the number of UTIs vs. controls.[202]

- Include yogurt, kefir, or sauerkraut in your diet to naturally support kidney health, strengthen immunity, and improve digestive balance.

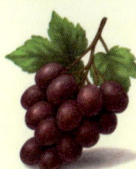

Resveratrol (Grape Skin Extract)

Resveratrol, found in red grape skins, blueberries, and other dark fruits, supports heart and kidney health by reducing inflammation, oxidative stress, and improving metabolism, making it potentially beneficial in protecting against chronic kidney disease.

- Aim for 150–500 mg/day of supplement or eat resveratrol-rich foods.

- A study in diabetics with kidney disease found 500 mg resveratrol lowered protein in urine and inflammation.[203]

- Skip red wine—resveratrol levels are low, and the alcohol may place added stress on the kidneys and overall detox systems.

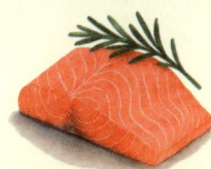

Salmon

Fatty fish like salmon, mackerel, and sardines are rich in omega-3 fatty acids (EPA and DHA). These healthy fats reduce inflammation, support blood vessel function, and may help protect kidney health, overall cardiovascular wellness, brain function, joint mobility, immune response, and metabolic balance.

- Aim for 8 oz of fatty fish per week (2 servings).

- 1,000 mg/day fish oil in dialysis patients reduced inflammation and slightly lowered creatinine.[204]

- If you don't eat fish, consider algae-based omega-3 supplements as a plant-based alternative to support heart, brain, and eye health.

Renal Support

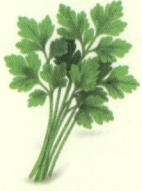

Parsley

Parsley contains flavonoids and volatile oils with antioxidant, anti-inflammatory, and mild diuretic effects. It helps flush waste, reduce bloating, and protect kidney tissue from damage.

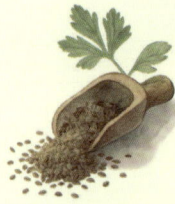

Celery Seed

Celery seed is a natural diuretic that helps eliminate excess fluids and ease pressure on the kidneys. Its phthalides and flavonoids support kidney health and reduce inflammation.

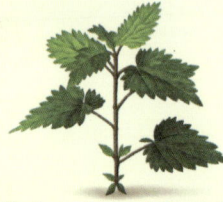

Stinging Nettle Root

Nettle root may lower DHT and estrogen levels while supporting free testosterone. It helps ease urinary symptoms such as weak flow, urgency, and frequent nighttime urination.

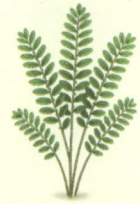

Chanca Piedra

Chanca piedra supports kidney health by breaking down and preventing the formation of stones. It also provides anti-inflammatory and antibacterial protection for the urinary tract and kidneys.

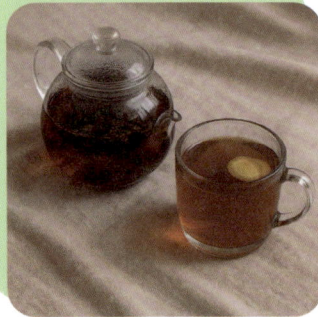

Herbal Kidney Cleanse Tea

This herbal kidney cleanse tea supports overall renal health with ingredients like bearberry leaf, hibiscus, and nettle leaf—herbs that act as natural diuretics to flush toxins, reduce inflammation, and promote healthy urine flow, easing the kidneys' workload.

Ingredients:
- 1 tsp dried bearberry leaf
- 1 tsp dried hibiscus
- 1 tsp dried nettle leaf
- 1-2 slices of ginger (optional)
- 1-2 cups hot water
- Honey (optional)

Instructions:
1. Boil water and add the dried herbs (bearberry leaf, hibiscus, and nettle leaf) to a tea infuser or directly into the water.
2. Let steep for 10-15 minutes.
3. Strain the herbs, add ginger slices (if using), and honey for sweetness.
4. Enjoy a warming kidney-supportive tea!

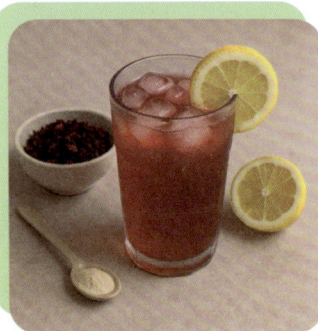

Resveratrol & Hibiscus Lemonade

This lemonade supports overall health because resveratrol is a powerful antioxidant that promotes heart and kidney function, while hibiscus helps lower blood pressure and supports the kidneys by acting as a natural diuretic and reducing oxidative stress.

Ingredients:
- 1 tbsp dried hibiscus flowers
- 1/2 tsp resveratrol powder
- 2 cups water
- Juice of 1 lemon
- 1 tbsp honey or stevia (optional)

Instructions:
1. Bring water to a boil and steep hibiscus flowers for 5-7 minutes.
2. Strain the flowers and let the liquid cool.
3. Stir in lemon juice and resveratrol powder.
4. Sweeten with honey or stevia to taste.
5. Serve chilled with ice cubes for a refreshing, kidney-supportive beverage.

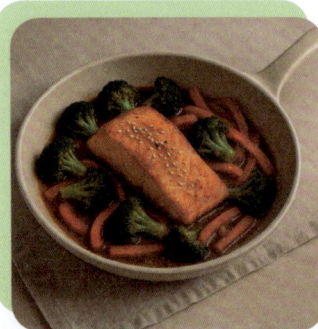

Salmon & Cordyceps Mushroom Stir-Fry

This stir-fry supports overall renal health because salmon is rich in omega-3s, which reduce kidney inflammation and support blood pressure, while cordyceps mushrooms are known to enhance kidney function, improve energy metabolism, and protect against oxidative stress.

Ingredients:
- 1 fatty fish fillet (e.g., salmon or mackerel)
- 1 tbsp olive oil
- 1/2 tsp cordyceps mushroom powder
- 1/2 cup broccoli florets
- 1/4 cup sliced bell peppers
- 1 tbsp low-sodium soy sauce
- 1 tsp sesame seeds (optional)

Instructions:
1. Sauté fish in olive oil until cooked.
2. Add broccoli and bell peppers; cook until tender.
3. Stir in cordyceps powder and soy sauce.
4. Top with sesame seeds and serve.

UTI Support

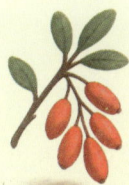

Berberine

Berberine is a plant alkaloid with strong antimicrobial effects. It helps prevent recurring UTIs by targeting harmful bacteria and supporting urinary tract health.

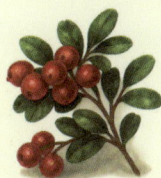

Lingonberry

Lingonberries contain PACs that prevent bacteria like *E. coli* from sticking to urinary tract walls. This promotes flushing during urination, reduces infection risk, and supports urinary tract health.

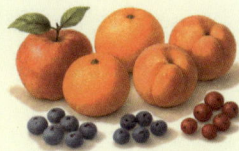

D-Mannose

D-mannose is a natural sugar that binds to *E. coli* and prevents it from attaching to the bladder. It helps flush bacteria out, supports UTI prevention, and promotes overall urinary tract health.

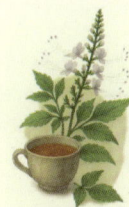

Java Tea (Orthosiphon stamineus)

Java tea contains flavonoids like rosmarinic acid that block bacterial adhesion in the bladder. This helps clear pathogens and lower the risk of UTIs.

Cranberry & Blueberry Smoothie

This smoothie is good for UTI prevention and kidney health because cranberries contain proanthocyanidins that help prevent bacteria from sticking to the urinary tract, while blueberries offer antioxidants that support kidney function and reduce inflammation.

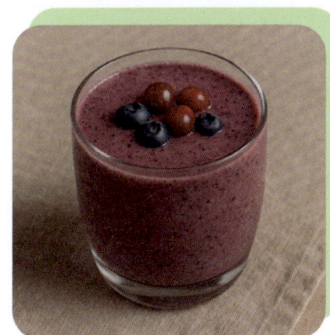

Ingredients:

- 1/2 cup fresh cranberries
- 1/2 cup fresh or frozen blueberries
- 1 cup unsweetened almond milk (or any preferred milk)
- 1 tbsp extra virgin olive oil (for healthy fats)
- 1 tbsp ground flaxseeds or chia seeds (optional for added fiber)
- 1/2 cup probiotic yogurt
- 1/2 tsp resveratrol powder (optional)

Instructions:

1. In a blender, combine cranberries, blueberries, almond milk, and olive oil.
2. Blend until smooth.
3. Add yogurt for probiotics and blend again.
4. Optionally, sprinkle in resveratrol powder for added antioxidant power.
5. Serve chilled and enjoy!

Probiotic & Chanca Piedra Yogurt Parfait

This parfait is good for UTIs because probiotics help maintain healthy gut and urinary tract flora, preventing harmful bacteria from thriving, while Chanca Piedra is traditionally used to support urinary tract health and may help reduce infection risk and kidney stones.

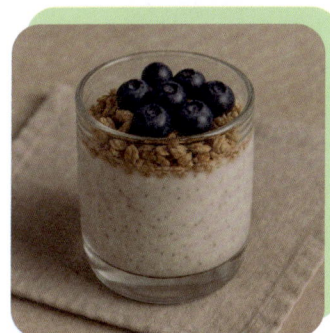

Ingredients:

- 1 cup probiotic yogurt
- 1/2 tsp Chanca Piedra powder
- 1/4 cup granola (optional)
- 1/4 cup fresh blueberries or lingonberries
- 1 tsp honey or maple syrup (optional)

Instructions:

1. Layer yogurt with Chanca Piedra powder in a small jar or glass.
2. Add granola and fresh berries for added texture and flavor.
3. Drizzle with honey or syrup (optional).
4. Enjoy as a snack that supports kidney health and digestion.

Iced Blueberry Matcha

Blueberries are rich in antioxidants and support kidney health by reducing inflammation and oxidative stress. Matcha provides gentle energy and is high in catechins, which help protect kidney cells and promote overall detoxification and balance.

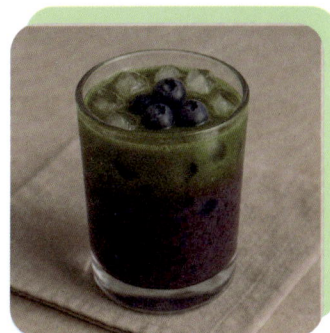

Ingredients:

- 1 tsp matcha powder
- ½ cup blueberries
- 1 tsp honey or stevia (optional)
- 1½ cups water
- ½ cup ice
- Splash of almond or oat milk (optional)
- Pinch of cinnamon (optional)

Instructions:

1. Blend blueberries with water; strain if desired.
2. Whisk matcha with warm water until smooth.
3. Combine all ingredients in a glass or shaker.
4. Add ice and milk (optional), stir or shake, and serve.

Bonus Tips

Daily Healing Habits & Routines

Small, consistent actions can lead to big, lasting changes in your wellness. Incorporate these simple habits into your daily life:

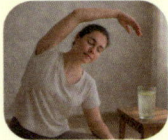

Morning Rituals

Start your day by hydrating with warm lemon water to kickstart digestion and hydrate your body. Follow with stretching to release tension and set a positive intention for the day ahead.

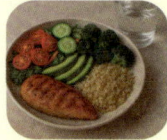

Balanced Meals

Fuel your body with whole foods, healthy fats, fiber, and clean protein. Minimize processed sugar and artificial additives to maintain stable energy and support overall health.

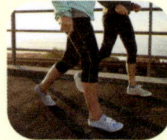

Movement

Even just 20 minutes of walking or light exercise boosts circulation, lymphatic flow, and mood. Find movement that works for you and make it part of your daily routine.

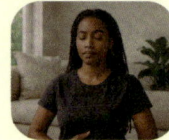

Mindfulness

Practice breathwork, journaling, or meditation for a few minutes each day to stay grounded and reduce stress. This enhances mental clarity and emotional balance.

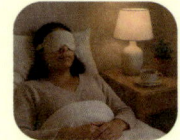

Sleep Hygiene

Stick to a consistent bedtime and reduce screen time at night. Create a calming bedtime routine to promote restful, rejuvenating sleep.

Essential Mind-Body Self-Care Practices

Nurturing your emotional and energetic well-being is crucial for overall health. Incorporate these practices into your daily or weekly routine to support balance and resilience:

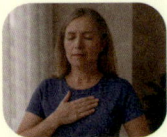

Breathwork

Practice deep belly breathing or alternate nostril breathing to activate the parasympathetic nervous system and reduce stress.

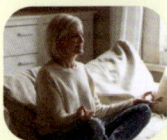

Meditation

Even five minutes of quiet reflection can reset your mindset, improve focus, and promote mental clarity.

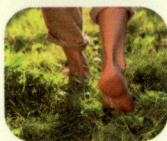

Grounding

Walk barefoot outdoors to reconnect with the Earth's energy, reducing stress and fostering a sense of calm.

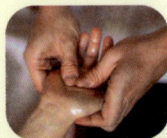

Acupressure

Stimulate specific pressure points on the body to alleviate tension, support organ function, and restore balance.

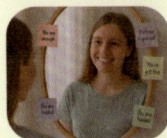

Affirmations or Visualization

Use positive affirmations or visualization techniques to align your thoughts with your healing intentions and goals.

Top 10 Remedies Every Home Needs

1. **Ginger**
Soothes nausea, aids digestion, and provides cold relief.

2. **Elderberry Syrup**
Boosts the immune system and has antiviral properties.

3. **Activated Charcoal**
Detoxifies, relieves food poisoning, and alleviates gas.

4. **Calendula Salve**
Heals skin, cuts, and rashes naturally.

5. **Chamomile Tea**
Promotes relaxation, aids digestion, and is great for children.

6. **Epsom Salt**
Relieves muscle tension and supports detox baths.

7. **Peppermint Oil**
Eases headaches, congestion, and muscle pain.

8. **Apple Cider Vinegar**
Improves digestion, balances pH, and soothes sore throats.

9. **Arnica Cream**
Reduces bruising, sprains, and muscle soreness.

10. **Raw Honey**
Fights coughs, speeds wound healing, and has antimicrobial properties.

Bonus Tips

Natural Healing First Aid Kit Essentials

Be prepared for minor emergencies with these natural, effective remedies that promote healing and comfort:

1. Lavender Essential Oil
Soothes stress, calms burns, and acts as a natural antiseptic for skin irritations.

2. Tea Tree Oil
Powerful antifungal and antibacterial oil, ideal for treating cuts, bites, and infections.

3. Rescue Remedy (Flower Essence)
A quick emotional support remedy to ease stress, shock, or trauma during a crisis.

4. Witch Hazel
Relieves skin irritations, reduces swelling, and can soothe hemorrhoids.

5. Slippery Elm Lozenges
Natural relief for sore throats and digestive discomfort.

6. Bentonite Clay
A detoxifying poultice for bug bites, skin eruptions, and drawing out toxins.

7. Comfrey Salve
Promotes healing for sprains, bruises, and even supports bone repair.

8. Bandages & Gauze
Essential for wound care and covering abrasions or cuts.

9. Thermometer & Tweezers
Basic tools for monitoring health and removing splinters or foreign objects.

Detox Rituals You Can Do at Home

Incorporating these simple, yet powerful rituals into your daily routine supports gentle detoxification and enhances your overall well-being:

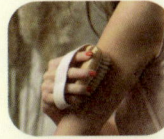

1. Dry Brushing
Stimulate lymphatic flow, exfoliate your skin, and promote circulation for a glowing complexion.

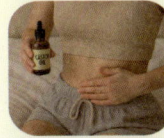

2. Castor Oil Packs
Applying warm castor oil to your abdomen as a pack may support relaxation, reduce bloating, and promote a sense of balance.

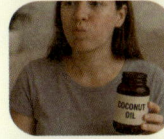

3. Oil Pulling
Swish coconut oil in your mouth for 10-15 minutes to draw out toxins, freshen breath, and promote oral health.

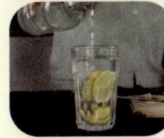

4. Hydration with Lemon Water
Start your day with a glass of lemon water to alkalize your body, boost digestion, and flush out toxins.

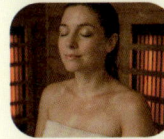

5. Infrared Sauna or Hot Baths
Induce sweating to help your body release toxins and relax your muscles, promoting overall detoxification.

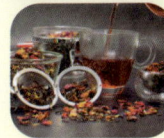

6. Herbal Teas
Enjoy detoxifying herbs like dandelion root, burdock, and nettle to support liver and kidney health while hydrating your body.

Seasonal Wellness Rituals

Aligning your self-care with the rhythms of nature can enhance balance and vitality year-round. Try these seasonal practices to stay grounded and nourished through every transition:

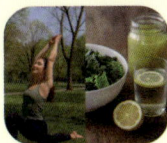

Spring
Gentle Cleanse

Support liver health with leafy greens, lemon water, and light movement like yoga or walking. Focus on renewal and decluttering.

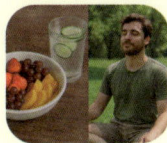

Summer
Cooling & Hydrating

Embrace fresh fruits, cucumber-infused water, and mint teas. Slow down, prioritize rest, and enjoy outdoor grounding.

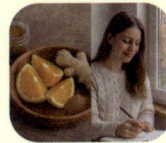

Autumn
Immune Support

Add warming spices like cinnamon and ginger, boost vitamin C, and start cozy rituals like journaling or early bedtimes.

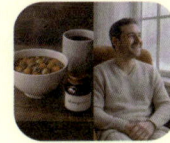

Winter
Deep Nourishment

Focus on hearty stews, adaptogenic herbs (like ashwagandha), and gentle self-reflection. Embrace warmth and inner stillness.

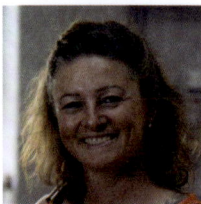

Introducing Shanon Greef

We're thrilled to introduce Shanon Greef, the insightful author behind our widely acclaimed green book, Ancient Remedies Revived. With a deep passion for natural wellness and traditional healing practices, Shanon has helped bring age-old wisdom back into the modern spotlight.

In addition to her solo work, she is also a proud co-contributor of The Natural Healing Handbook, where she continues to inspire readers with practical, holistic approaches to health and well-being. Her work bridges the gap between ancient knowledge and modern living; making natural healing both accessible and relevant today.

Revised Edition, September 2025